How to be a
Spiritual
Christian

(What Demons Don't Want You to Know)

by

Pastor/Exorcist Sharon L. Flesher

How to be a Spiritual Christian

Copyrighted 2009 by Sharon Flesher.

For information please direct your inquiries to:

Bread & Wine Ministries
7961 E. Hwy U
Eldorado Springs, MO. 64744
breadandwineministries@hotmail.com

ISBN: 978-09844893-0-5

This book is dedicated to my children....

Megan and Shannon for their unending patience, and to Ashley and Hunter for their everlasting hugs.

Contents

Snapshots

In him was life; and the life was the light of men

John 1:4 (KJV)

Foreword

I began this book with the intention of titling it *What Demons Don't Want you to Know* but as the book unfolded and revelations came I realized that the title was not adequate and it took second place to the importance of how much God loves His creation. I discovered, to my wondrous delight, a more in-depth understanding of His gentle nature, kind heart, and the mechanics behind the world we live in and rewrote my book accordingly. I realized that people needed to be able to connect with God in a special way and to understand how their world and spirit functions.

Yes, demons do play a significant role in the demise of humanity and it is covered extensively in this book, but there is something much deeper that lies at the root cause of the destruction of mankind's soul; a destruction aided by a force we cannot see.

What really surprised me was the way this book seem to unfold on its own before my very eyes. I was astounded and I hope you will be too. May your heart be drawn in an everlasting pull to the Creator of your soul; the gentle Spirit who never seems to tire with our failings. May we always stand in awe of His deep love for humanity whose compassion and mercy cannot be measured.

As you go through life you have come to know and realize that in your own spirit you are not alone. How many times have you caught yourself in a verbal conversation with someone who isn't there?

Just who is it that you argue with? Why do we always feel that there is more than one person with us all the time with whom we struggle? We are constantly justifying, excusing, arguing, blaming, and reasoning with our own 'selves'. There is a battle within of good and evil which is beyond our own presence and we feel it. Who can escape a guilty heart?

Often we are compelled to do things that we later on regret and find ourselves tormented from within. Where are these 'outside' emotions coming from, these minds that voice their opinions and seem to have little to no regard for our feelings? If you were truly your own person, why are you having trouble convincing yourself of things? If you don't want to be angry why don't you just stop? Have you ever tried to forget something that you wanted to forget? It just won't go away, will it? Deep down inside of us all we know there is a war going on.

We use many things to ease the pain of life, and then are forced to live with the consequences of the choices we made. Seeking refuge in alcohol, drugs, sex, television, video games, ambitions, goals, work, and even religion and we run from one distraction to the next. Anything that pulls us away from all that is going on inside of us we welcome with open arms.

Then, as the guilt compounds it develops into fear and from fear comes stress. The sins we entertain seem to thicken and adhere like tar upon our souls. The more we sin the more it takes to deaden the voices and the more we deaden the voices the guiltier we become which in turn makes the inner voices scream even louder. It's much like a tire on a steep slope, picking up speed as it travels faster and further down the hill. Eventually it is bound to reach the bottom in some disastrous form or another, and so goes the life of the human soul.

Where is your peace at? Where is true life? Can man really know His Maker and live in peace with Him?

This book is written with the intent of awakening you to the reality of the spirit world around you and in you and help you function as you were meant to. Therefore, the contents of this book will deeply disturb some and so I apologize in advance for any fear you will most likely experience as you learn the truth for yourself and also for anything else that may occur. It is much like being abruptly awaken during a deep sleep. You may feel a little disconnected to yourself and you also may get a sense of running, anger, or horror as you may well come face to face with Reality. If it should occur, just quietly hold your peace, it isn't you that feels this fear and panic, but the 'not you' with whom you contend. I pray that you have what it takes to hear the message in this book. If you do......it will change your life.

—Sharon

<u>One</u>

What is Spirituality?

Spirit verses matter.......

What does it mean to be spiritual? What is the difference between a spiritual person and a carnal person? We observe a defined difference in the behavior of people in and around the world. We know that there is right and wrong, good and bad, truth and lies. Is this what it means to be spiritual or nonspiritual? I would ask you this, "can anything be nonspiritual?" The answer is a defined, "no." For all things emanate and originate from the all Spirit God. Therefore, there can only be two spiritual paths to travel. A wrong spiritual path and a right spiritual path. The wrong path is often referred to as a carnal path because it is based upon the mind set that differs from Truth—from God's Mind.

How are we able to discern the difference in us? How is it that every human being appears to have a 'Mind' or 'Conscience' with similar and most often nearly identical convictions? Who tells us what is right and wrong? Who defines these differences to our understanding? It is the Creator, who made us,

He allows us to see and know. His Spirit resides within all mankind. Whether we listen and follow is certainly another issue.

So we see that that which we have understood as carnal is just another spiritual force that is present or the lack of our Creator's and we have falsely thought that the carnal mind was perhaps our own ignorance—namely ourselves. We have claimed to be all the noise and confusion within us supposing, perhaps in pride, that we argue with our own selves. If we are not even aware of the voices in us what about what is going on in the world around us. What does it consist of? Is matter that which is real or unreal? Are spirit and matter differing or opposing forces? Where did matter come from? Matter originated in and of Spirit, did it not? What you see as matter is only vibrations. Science has proven that if you take a powerful microscope you can see through anything that appears to be solid. It only feels solid because it is vibrating. Therefore it is entirely possible that if one could vibrate at the same level as matter you could truly walk through a wall. Did you know that I know of people have done that and practice it today? I tell you the truth and by the end of this book you may grasp a basic understanding of its possibility and hopefully you will also understand how you are creating your own world by and through your own vibrations—unbeknownst to you. Not because you are God with mighty powers and such, as you are not, but because God ordained your world to function in a particular

2

way; a way, so far, that you have not seen. You see, this world is operating on and by His Spiritual Laws and these laws are in effect whether we comprehend them or not.

By the time you get to the end of this book you will discover why things do or don't work out for you and why a person is either blessed or cursed in what they do in life even down to the smallest of actions. Nothing is overlooked by God who is everywhere at once and knows everything.

What is matter? Matter is simply a product of spirit. It is most certainly real, as it exists in and of God. It is subject to Spirit and only exists within Him. Your matter, or the matter you live within, has become a product of your spirit/heart, the center of who you are and your own spirit creates the world around you. You are ever changing by the vibrations you are emitting. Just as God's Spirit hovered over the waters and made the world, your spirit hovers over your own life and body creating the world you live in today and the one you will have tomorrow. We are made in His image and operate as He does. What you are on the inside is soon to become your outside. (*Your heart will soar when you realize that these things never change and that justice is more than alive.*) Seeing that matter is spirit, matter then cannot be absence of Spirit or not real. The truth is that spirituality and carnality are levels of complex vibrations on two wave lengths, levels, or perimeters. You are either from above or beneath in all that you do and only one has your allegiance.

3

A spiritual Christian is a misnomer for all who are born of Spirit are indeed spiritual. In truth all people are spiritual as all matter is a product of spirit. Even those who are carnally minded are following spirits and spiritually led. I chose the title of this book for the concept behind it. I knew in my heart that only those who really want more of God would want to be a 'spiritual' Christian. All who truly love God wish to be closer and more 'spiritually minded' rather than 'earthly minded', therefore, I hope that I am reaching ears that will listen to truth.

God is the 'all Spirit God' and all that you see, including yourself, came from Him and exists in Him by his origin and design. His Spirit is the source behind all vibrations. Therefore matter is real, but not in the sense that mankind has first understood it to be, but rather it is set to vibrate by His Spirit to feel solid to our own spirits and according to the frequencies/oscillations that we vibrate upon. Again, this is God's design. All creation is His thought manifest. Your life is and has become your thought manifest according to and in alignment with His spiritual laws. Again, all that you see is moving and operating according to His principals and laws. This is how God designed it to be. I will expound upon these spiritual laws and principals that you and I live within as we go along. You will be astounded as you see that you are indeed becoming your thoughts.

Science has also proven that every thought has a

frequency. You are spirit. You are a vibrational creature. Your body is also vibration but corrupted and must be recreated one day to the correct frequency/vibration/oscillation in order to dwell in harmony with God. This uncorrupted body is called a glorified body in the bible and will not have corrupted frequencies and vibrations.

The religions that teach matter as not real, may have meant that it wasn't solid or as it appeared. Keeping this in mind I move forward. Matter, therefore, is also spirit and is subject to it. They are not separate as taught by the world/low frequency minds. Matter is a product of Spirit vibrations. For lack of better words I'm going to refer to the vibrations as:

Low Frequency: LF>Incorrect thoughts, emotions, concepts, and ways... (carnal/earthly/worldly,flesh)

High Frequency: HF>Correct thoughts, emotions, concepts, and ways....
(Godly/heavenly/Holy/Spiritual).

The bible uses different ways to express the same theme of these frequencies. In this book we will take a look at them. Basically, the higher your frequencies the more in line you are with your Creator. The lower you vibrate, the more out of line you are with Him and the closer you are to death (little to no vibration).

Mankind use to have higher vibrations, but the

moment Adam moved upon a low frequency thought, he fell. He was then removed from the garden of Eden (pure dimension/vibrations) to the earth (corrupt frequencies and vibrations) and immediately entered death in his spirit. We are now low vibrational creatures. To be saved, you have to be reborn in spirit to high frequencies. This can only come about through repentance which is a sincere turning from low frequency thoughts and emotions to high ones.

I know this isn't emotionally satisfying to hear. The emotional high one gets from joining a secret club of special people who have magic words and special club names like 'Presbyterian or Lutheran' are of the flesh, not God. This book is a book of Truth and was given to me by Divine Revelation and is not written to pacify the flesh. The religious will not like this book. I hope you are not one of them but a seeker of Truth.

9 For as the heavens are higher than the earth, so are my ways higher than your ways, and my thoughts than your thoughts.   Isaiah 55:9 (KJV)

The Creators ways are all High Frequency. Every thought and emotion that He emits is correct. He has no low vibrational thoughts and ways that He moves upon. He is fully aware of evil, having made that frequency range, just as a person is aware that he casts a shadow, but it is not who He is, nor is defined by or through it.

6

15 Who is the image of the invisible God, the firstborn of every creature:

16 For by him were all things created, that are in heaven, and that are in earth, visible and invisible, whether they be thrones, or dominions, or principalities, or powers: all things were created by him, and for him:

17 And he is before all things, and by him all things consist.

Col 1:16-17 (KJV)

(Also, please don't skip over the scriptures in this book and read them slowly and let them sink in as they contain deeper revelations if viewed with my writings. Some of you --those with the gift of Wisdom-- will be able to see an even deeper revelation of this book if you move slowly and read them together....if your mind feels full, stop, reflect, and return when you feel hungry again....thank you for dining gracefully upon the bread of Christ.)

If God, who is all and in all, is pure Spirit how can there be anything but Spirit? There isn't. Remember we already know that all creation, all matter, is simply a vibration. All that you see, feel, smell, hear, and touch are vibrations. Your brain is receiving all that it knows through these oscillations and vibrations. Therefore, we can easily see that matter is simply a product of Spirit and is subject to it.

Matter can absolutely affect matter. Rain for instance can touch dirt and create mud. Poison ingested can kill you. Healthy food will help create a healthy body and there is wisdom in eating right. One of God's laws or principalities that he created was that matter affects matter. You can most certainly move within this law and bring much goodness or harm into your life.

Next, we see a higher law. In this law Spirit effects matter. This law overrides the lower law. It really is 'Mind over matter'. For instance, a healthy person can become sick from worry. Here we see that vibrations from your own spirit can immediately affect the body. Long and short term effects come from both HF and LF thoughts depending on the severity of either one.

Everything you see has Spirit in it. All creation, even rocks have Spirit in them, for God is all and therefore is matter itself. But not all spirit filled objects are given equal Consciences or abilities. When you sit on a rock, you are sitting on a piece of Him. His vibrations are moving in that rock to keep it there for you to sit on. You are allowed to split it, crush it, or use it. He doesn't mind. As long as you are 'lawful' with His creation. This means that as long as you move within His boundaries of usage with His matter there is no sin involved in how you treat Him as Creation. However, should you break off a piece of stone and smash someone in the head with it, you will be held accountable. This is 'unlawful' use of His creation, not to mention how you treated your fellow man. All creation exists within His laws. There are differing kinds of spirits with differing laws. The earth has a spirit. It cries out and creation worships God and has a different kind of spirit than human beings.

39 All flesh *is* not the same flesh: but *there is* one *kind of* flesh of men, another flesh of beasts, another of fishes, *and* another of birds.

All low frequencies are not the same. They are on differing levels with differing consciences. Every frequency has a 'kind'. We are not animals nor have we ever come from an animal. Animals can kill. It is lawful for them to do so, but not to kill people. These are corrupt animals and are punished by God. Therefore, we see that even animals can become corrupt and move on LF thoughts (Gen. 1:12). Mankind has a higher conscience and is held to a higher standard. Animals can become corrupt as well as humans and are able to move outside of its lawful design. Once it does so, it is condemned and cannot return into harmony with its Creator.

40 *There are* also celestial bodies, and bodies terrestrial: but the glory of the celestial *is* one, and the *glory* of the terrestrial *is* another.

Each of God's creation began as a different

thought anchored to a picture in God's Mind which is why all creation is good and wondrous. Remember, every thought has a frequency, even God's, and each creation is on a different wave length or scale (for lack of better words) and what you see described in Genesis is a projection of God's mind coming to pass. The earth was lowered in frequency once the thoughts in creation became corrupted and man was moved from the garden of Eden to a place of death and destruction. This is how all bad things come into your own life. The lower your frequency the more you will enter cursings/death.

41 *There is* one glory of the sun, and another glory of the moon, and another glory of the stars: for *one* star differeth from *another* star in glory.
1 Cor 15:38-41 (KJV)

Even the stars have their own vibrations just as every snowflake, every speck of sand, and every hair on everyone's head in the world. God knows them all and is acutely aware of every particle of His own being. We are His thoughts and what He doesn't wish to think about will soon be forgotten. This is eternal hell. All who partake will suffer his everlasting indignation which will be highly unpleasant.

No part of God can become missing which is why you will exist somewhere forever. He is all. If you were to take away from all, it wouldn't be all now would it? Therefore, all that you think you have lost, never was and you are already healed by His stripes because all that you see has already been before. All things are in and of Him. Things that seem to be displaced such as lost loved ones, the house that use to be new, and your things, these only move from one vibration to another as it is moved from one place in Him to another. Guess what that means? Your childhood was never gone. It is complete in Him. He is the data base and can bring back anything he desires at anytime anywhere. These are His storehouses. You are His thought. He has a folder He calls 'The book of Life'. Here the names of HF transmitters are recorded.

Science has already noticed that energy is never gone. It is always moving. Things rot, grow, rot, and grow. God is pure Energy and can never be diluted or lessened. One can never lose Him. All things are in Him and of Him and the earth and stars are all moving by His power and design and is complete in Him....lacking nothing.

6 **By the word of the LORD were the heavens made; and all the host of them by the breath of his mouth.**

7 **He gathereth the waters of the sea together as an heap: he layeth up the depth in storehouses.**

8 **Let all the earth fear the LORD: let all the**

inhabitants of the world stand in awe of him.

Psalms 33:5-8 (KJV)

And in awe we should be. God has storehouses or places in Him, like a thought not quite brought about that holds many things. He can bring frogs, locusts, lice, rain, or hail at will.....we are after all....just a product of His thinking. Just as your soul is a product of your own thinking, our world, spirit, and all existence is a product of His. This is what He meant when He said we were made in His image. We function on a smaller level as He does. He creates with thought and so do we. Our Spirits function like His with one huge difference....His thoughts are all correct and all that He does is good, perfect, and just. His thoughts are all perfect in intent and application. We have much to learn. What if we refuse to do so?

To be a spiritual Christian is to be a person whose mind, ways, emotions, and thoughts are of God and seeking God (higher vibrations). To really have Jesus as the Lord of your life means that you are putting all that is right and good and true first place in your heart because you love Him/Truth. You became a new creature in Christ when you cried out to be delivered from the low frequency/sin in your life. The glorious presence of the guiding Light, the Holy Spirit, shown brightly in your inner man and you saw your sin! You became aware of your wrong thinking and you turned to Him and cried out to be delivered—you believed. The Truth changed you from a creature who was lost and loved the dark, to a creature of the Light. You gave your heart to God/Truth and turned from sin/wrong thinking.

Your enemy is wrong thinking, emotions, and low frequencies. Yes, unclean spirits aid humanity in its demise, but they only move within our wrong thinking—our sin. Satan is the one who fathers or nurtures all wrong thinking in this world. He is not the source of evil as he did not create it but he father's those who love it. Therefore, to be spiritual, as in Godly spiritual, you must come up from the darkness and enter the Light and God will then move through you and keep you. You must become a child of Light instead of a child of darkness as you once were. God isn't into preserving sin(wrong thinking acted on) and sinners so if you move from thoughts that aren't His He isn't going to be there to back them or you up. Your real enemy is the same one that Jesus had, the devil, and you will destroy him just as Jesus did— with the Truth.

Those who view the physical as that which is real and use it to verify that which is spiritual are looking at Reality in a reverse way. It would be the equivalent of examining a cake to figure out what a stove and baker were. The cake has little to do with who made it other then it was good and reflects the ability and mentality of the person who made it. Instead of realizing that behind every cake is an oven and a baker people tend to think that everything came from and consists of cake.

God, Spirit, created all that you see and so that which is physical has originated from that which is invisible. For those who try to explain and discover the invisible with the physical they find constant frustration for though they try, there are many things in this world that contradict the physical senses. Just as one realizes a cake cannot appear from no where, so we all know that life has to come from some place. We invented several stories in an attempt to solve the reality that the cake didn't bake itself but even our super computers say that theories such as Evolution are simply impossible. Looking at the complexity of creation, deep down inside we know and understand that there is indeed a Creator and we are here by super intelligent design. So Reality begins in Him and is Him. Creation, the physical world we see, is simply a manifestation from the Creator Himself.

Scientist generally turn away from the evidence of the spirit world and instead work to disprove it. Is that real science? No, it is man with a hidden agenda and when you go at anything with a preconceived notion it is not science but deception funded by bureaucracy; two evils set on a course for hell's fire.

Remember, God isn't just 'a' spirit....He is 'the' Spirit. He is the source of all life. All things consist in and of Him.

Two

Negative and Positive Energy

Understanding their function in Creation....

What is negative energy? Is it a force unto itself doing and moving at its own will? The answer is yes and no. Let me explain.

All power is God's therefore negative energy did not come into existence by some outside force as there is none. God, in His wisdom, has given and set up dominions and principalities. Negative energy is one of these powers.

16 **For by him were all things created, that are in heaven, and that are in earth, visible and invisible, whether** *they be* **thrones, or dominions, or principalities, or powers: all things were created by him, and for him:**

17 **And he is before all things, and by him all things consist.**

Col 1:16-17 (KJV)

Therefore, negative energy is a real power and operates on LF and is designed to give all creation a choice between the force of good or evil. You can either follow thoughts and ways that He approves of or thoughts and ways he disapproves of. He wants sons and daughters, not robots and is in the process of creating children.

Negative energy can be viewed as the lack of Positive energy. Positive energy is Unity with God. When your spirit aligns with His then He flows through you. Therefore positive energy can only come from speaking and moving upon Truth. Man is complex in that his emotion, will, intent, and intellect must align in order to unify with the Creator.

Positive confessions and affirmations are only those that align with the Truth. All affirmations made in the flesh are not positive, though they may sound like it to wanton ears.

The force behind negative energy, what is it? It is the realm of the dark and all LF creatures that dwell there. This encapsulates such creatures as satan, devils, unclean spirits, demons, and people that love these spirits.

What is the force behind positive energy? The Holy Spirit, which is God's own spirit, Angels, and anyone who is moving from God's Spirit are those who are Him and with Him in the earth.

Is it possible to move from positive and negative energy? Absolutely! Paul told us to have a person with the gift of discernment stand present when people prophesied. Why? A person can easily come from a wrong place in their heart and speak for other spirits.

What are we? We are spirit. All is Spirit. We pick up frequencies much like a radio. Whatever station you tune into, you transmit. This is why Jesus said that Peter spoke for God through revelation one minute and then He promptly turned and rebuked satan in Peter the next. We simply transmit and we hear from the spirit we come from.

What is the secret to hearing and moving from God? A pure heart. For only the pure in heart see God (Matt. 5:8). Therefore your task in the earth is to destroy the devil in you. It isn't to become more than anyone else, for God is all. Your race, your task, your problems originate within your own heart and soul. Pride has many struggles seeing this and I will expound upon it as we go along.

The demonic realm does pull at your soul but they can only affect the areas of your life that are already corrupt. Once you have made the initial turn from LF, cried out to God by believing that Jesus died for your LF and you give your life to Him, to live unto HF the war is on! You are now in a full front battle with the enemy. Before, you were moving smoothly along with the enemy of God, thinking his thoughts, moving upon his ways, and being an extension of darkness in the earth. Let's take a closer look at the forces of darkness. Who are they, how are they able to reach you and use you?

I've heard it said that if you want to catch a crook

you have to think like one. Understanding how Satan, unclean spirits, demons, and the people they use think and move will help you understand what a low frequency thought is, how to evade them, and why the message of 'who' unclean spirits are appears to be missing from the bible today. Once you begin to see their pattern of thoughts and ways it will help you to separate from them. It is important to understand the forces behind sin (wrong thinking acted on) and to understand how death, cursings, and destruction are entering your life in order for you to quit moving upon them; sending out corrupt vibrations. Just who is it that helps us into wrong thoughts and emotion misleading us from the way of Life?

Who did Jesus find at fault for the sicknesses and demise of humanity? Who did He come against to heal people and set them free and who did He hold responsible for their deaths, sicknesses, and tormenting situations. What force/energy is behind a cursed life?

17 And he (Jesus) **came down with them, and stood in the plain, and the company of his disciples, and a great multitude of people out of all Judaea and Jerusalem, and from the sea coast of Tyre and Sidon, which came to hear him, and to be healed of their diseases; 18 And they that were vexed with unclean spirits: and they were healed.**

Luke 6:17-18 (KJV)

The people came to hear the Truth and to be healed. Who is vexing the people? Right, unclean spirits. These are those voices that argue in your head and lead you astray. These are those who come to steal, kill, and destroy your life. Jesus knew that they must hear the Truth and receive it to be well. However, the unclean spirit had to also be removed. Now, seeing that such a great enemy is at hand, let me ask you this...... who are they, how are they able to attack you, and how can you stop them? Surely in such an age with so many many churches and so much religion such a simple question should have been answered correctly by now. It has not nor has it drawn full attention of those who claim to be spiritual Christian leaders. Why? Could it be the unclean spirits themselves working through religious leaders and others in a quest to stay hidden? Yes, unclean spirits campaign *heavily* to stay hidden from people's view and for the most part it has worked, hasn't it? Even though they are super active in every person you know, including yourself, most cannot see them or detect them. You see, the quality of the unclean spirits lives depend upon your ignorance as they destroy you to live.

(People often find the truth of what I know highly uncomfortable for various reasons and so I am forewarning you that this book will move you well out of your comfort zone. Brace yourself, you are about to meet Reality.)

I'm hopeful that you are wise enough to listen to my words and receive them to your benefit. It is human nature to abandon what is not pleasant to him, this causes him to lose sight of the truth as the truth tends to bring discomfort to the areas in our hearts that are not correct. Generally, people don't want to know anything that they do not perceive as advantageous to their already established religions, philosophies, and egos (false images of themselves).

How many times has the truth been discarded for what was more pleasant to the soul? We throw God out the window to keep the devils and wonder why things go wrong in our lives. Keeping this in mind, please realize that what you perceive has nothing to do with Reality. Reality isn't changed by our perception. It remains in tact as a whole regardless of what we choose to see or not see. I am simply stating that human beings tend to see only what they want to see; regardless of how things really are. Deception begins in the heart and once accepted it, like yeast, permeates our entire beings and lives. Here, in us, it lives and grows and seeks to enter others so it can grow there too. All who knowingly and lovingly practice deception cannot be lovers of Truth or fathered by Him, can they?

Speaking of deception, who is the biggest deceiver? What creature is the biggest liar? We've all told a few in our lifetime, right? Okay, honestly probably more then a few...however, who is the biggest liar of us all? I'm sure you have a particular person in mind and probably a family member or someone you've spent extended time with that has successfully conned you on a continual basis but they are all losers compared to Satan. The bible calls Satan the 'father of lies' (John 8:44) as he successfully conned Adam and Eve and brought us into a lie loving world. Satan, the serpent, is still active today through all who love and practice lies. He is not omnipresent so how is he able to do that? We will look into that process in greater detail in a moment, but for now I would like to point out that God 'cannot' lie (Titus 1:2). The reason why is that to 'lie' is a sin (wrong thinking acted on) and God is sinless; without even one wrong or incorrect piece of data in Him. Therefore, He cannot lie. He cannot emit a low frequency thought to move upon. He is Truth. It is actually impossible for Him to lie. In the Truth there cannot be nor is there anything that is incorrect. No lies are ever present in absolute Truth. **He is absolute Truth— High Frequency. This is who He is.**

All unclean spirits and evil spirits lie. They simply cannot help it, it is who they are and what they do. It is how they got to where they are at and why they are still there. They loved their own imagination above Reality. You will see later on, as I get into more details, why this simple truth is of such great importance. Demons lie and lie through people and Satan teaches them as he is the lowest frequency—most corrupt. All low frequency thoughts are based upon that which is not true which is why God does not think as they do nor are His emotions like theirs.

There are many 'bragging' ministries out there concerning demonic expulsion, but very few who really know what they are talking about concerning demons and demonology. This is because demonic spirits are helping them go astray and they are not aware of it and I'm not saying that to demean them. It is just a fact. One can only move upon the truth that one is willing to accept or that one has present in one's heart. When you realize that the main opinion that the church has of the demonic realm is based almost entirely upon conjecture and assumptions, not scripture or the understanding of spirits that those who walked in the days of Jesus possessed, you will see that the false doctrine of Nephilims and fallen angels as unclean spirits is not even close to being scriptural or correct. Why do so many religions back it so fervently? Who is teaching them to lie and prodding them onto and into their false theology? Is this the Holy Spirit, who cannot lie? Probably not. Then just who is behind the scenes of the theologians, pushing their pens, and talking in their ears to give them such knowledge? Could it be unclean spirits themselves, protecting their own kingdoms, their homes, and their way of life? When is the last time you heard a preacher tell you where and how an unclean spirit lives, works, and moves and then expound upon how it is able to enter, fool you, and destroy your life? Seeing that Jesus made such a point to deliver people from them, shouldn't we pay heed and do as

He did? Where is the information to let you know how they make you sick, and kill you? Who is hiding it from you and why?

Stealth is one of the demon's biggest weapon. You can't destroy, fight, or overcome what you do not know exists can you? Unclean spirits are very active in everyone's lives. Can you detect them? If not, why? An unclean spirit tempts you often and the bible says they do and lets you know it is an everyday affair.

7 Submit yourselves therefore to God. Resist the devil, and he will flee from you.

James 4:7 (KJV)

An unclean spirit may tell you a bit of truth to make their lie seem real, but in the end—it was a lie. It is exactly the way that Satan beguiled Eve. All good lies are nearly ninety-nine percent true and the best lies are always the most 'believable' ones and all are based upon your misguided desires. Every salesman knows that the product they sell must have some plausibility to be believed and some enticing aspect to be bought. So it is with you and I, demons know that you must buy the lie to sell the lie. They can only live within lies in us as they are low frequency vibrations. So what is your real enemy? Is it the demon? No, they are just the salesmen..... it's the corruption in your own heart. It is your own sins that you move from that get in your way and keep you from God—the kingdom of heaven. Demons reinforce what is *already* incorrect in you. They can only survive in the places in your life where you vibrate on low frequency. Therefore, people die from a lack of knowledge (high frequencies) Hos. 4:6.

One thing that I also need to clarify early on, is that not all demons are unclean spirits. Unclean spirits are the main spirits that enter people. They are the ones that generally possess people, make people sick, and the ones we contend with on a daily basis. Unclean spirits are unclean because they have not been 'cleansed' by the Word of God/Truth. Their frequencies are impure which is why they are unclean. They are not spirits that can dwell in unity with the Truth and therefore are apart from Him. The spirit that leads them and teaches them lies is Satan or Lucifer, the father of all liars. God has designed creation this way for a reason. He is making sons and daughters and His children must be able to choose between life or death; right and wrong. It is not His will that any should perish and know that low frequencies would exist regardless of whether people thought them or not. Like I said before, evil is merely the shadow of God. It is made by Him but does not hold his attributes nor his emotions or thoughts.

Satan is not an unclean spirit and is not omnipresent. He vibrates the furthest from God as he is the furthest from the Truth which is why to be a great satanist you have to break all of the ten commandments and only the most morbid of men can invoke him. If you are a satanist and have not truly met Satan yet, know that you must lower your frequencies and destroy any (HF) in you that might exist as all HF is detestable to Satan. You will be demonically possessed in the process but you will be allowed to think you are making all the decisions in your life for a time. You will succumb to Satan one revelation (believable lie) at a time until you are wholly evil—wholly his. Liars are the first to hit the eternal flames (Rev. 21:8) as they are the furthest from the Truth. To be a full blown satanist you cannot have truth, love, or goodness in your heart. These are all HF vibrations.

Who is Satan? The bible says that Satan wasn't a human but that he was a seraphim and that he was a worshiping angel named Lucifer (Isa. 14:12). He was seen in the garden as a dragon or seraphim, lost his legs and is described as a serpent in Revelations. Evil's existence in our world is aided by evil people but is not dependent on them or Satan. Evil/LF was in existence long before Satan came along.

Satan is just the first creature in our dimension to fall therefore he is the most corrupt. He fell in love with himself and sought to be God. Many people think that Satan is human like them or in a humanoid form. He is not. He basically looks or looked like a dragon or a type of dinosaur who lost his legs in the garden of Eden to become the serpent. The bible also calls him Leviathan (Rev. 20:2). The point here is that God made him extremely wise and beautiful, even so much that he fell in love with himself and saw his 'own' goodness apart from God, not of God, but separate from Him and belonging to himself.....hence he became a lie lover, as God is all and in all. This root character will be behind every person who has gone astray or is going astray from Truth/God and is the bond of all low frequencies emitters. Once you 'adore' yourself and seek to be adored, you set all common sense and right thinking aside for the false reality you just 'made up' about your fake wonderful self and this pride, this love of self, is the root of all your failings. Satan's characteristics will be behind all lying and lie lovers who despise the Truth which is why he 'father's' or leads the lie lovers. For this reason Satan seems to be omnipresent because his character reigns in and throughout the spirits who have access to us.

God created good and evil which is the same as saying God created the light and darkness, high frequencies and low frequencies, right and wrong, truth and lies. All things are made with opposites by Him—God's very presence creates this effect. When we begin to move within high frequencies and we learn to move with Life, not against Him, struggling will cease, peace will be found, and salvation will be known in us and healing to the body comes naturally.

One way we struggle against Him is that we assume He has errors and sin in Him. Our false thinking causes us to believe that God is just a more powerful sinner than we are and so we set out to overcome Him just as we do others on earth. This thought process is taught to us by the spirits of this world, our parents, and the unregenerate minds that have access to us.

Evil spirits don't want you to know that God doesn't lie or sin and that in Him is no sin. This is one of their little dirty secrets. They like you to sympathize with Lucifer and those who sin and follow him and make Satan, yourself, and others out to be a victim of an unjust unfair Creator. Many secretly believe that Satan will also be saved one day, that it isn't his fault that he is evil, and that his goodness will one day be redeemed. Some people I know even feel sorry for him. Please realize that Satan was in God's presence, he saw 'all' the Truth and turned from it. How can there be an redemption or place to repent when there is nothing new to discover? This is why he is completely evil. There is no good in him. He left it all behind for love of the lie, for love of self. He fell from Heaven/High frequencies after emitting them and has no where to go to find repentance.

In order for any fall to take place one must have something to 'fall' from. So you will see that is the case in every situation where you are moving in LF. You either fell from the truth or you simply did not have the truth in the first place to move from and began in the lower frequencies; the fallen state. If the Truth was not present in your heart to move from what could you do? Before you ever fell into a sin it was because you believed it first, either from ignorance, lack of understanding, or rebellion to the truth; regardless, the lie/LF was chosen and moved upon. This today is the source of corruption in your life. You must find a way to unite your mind/spirit with God's in order to live as He is Life itself.

The way to salvation is easy to see. Just as in death one is united with Satan and LF, to live is to reverse the process. LF must be removed, but how? A person is not the source of HF or LF but only transmits. How can one move from the dark to the Light to be saved? Salvation is all about repentance, is it not? Repenting is where you see the truth in your inner man by the Light of God and through conviction, you turn from that which was not right to that which is right but you must do so by and within the inner man with sincere convictions.

When you have the Truth and move upon Him in you, then all the snares of the enemy are in vain. This is why safety is 'of the Lord/Truth'. Who can snatch you away from God....from Truth revealed to your inner man? No one. And no one ever falls into traps set in plain sight, do they?

Surely in vain the net is spread in the sight of any bird.   Prov 1:17 (KJV)

So it is our inability to see and accept the Truth in our lives that allows demonic spirits and lies to live and rule us thereby destroying us. One of their biggest weapons against you is to get you to doubt

28

the Truth, to doubt what you know is right by presenting an alternative to right that appeals to your ego. We usually begin to question the truth because it brings conflict to our lives or upsets our egos. We suddenly find ourselves at odds with those who love lies and struggle with our own lusts. Often we are not willing to suffer the consequences or bear the burden, our cross, that comes with knowing the truth. The 'other' truth, the one we concoct, becomes more pleasing to our egos and gets the approval of those who surround us in our every day lives. We begin to make excuses for our sin and blame others; standing in full denial. Having company with other sinners eases our guilt momentarily and we seek distractions to avoid having to hear our consciences. All corruption and spirit influence begins from and within your own heart and spirit. Have heart, this also means the cure lies in the same place.

It isn't theology, per-say that gets us in trouble but questioning those things that God has revealed to us through divine revelations within our own hearts. These are the talents that the bible speaks of that we will be accountable for in Matt. 25. When you doubt what you know is right and move on what you 'know' is incorrect to get something that you want for self advantage, that is when you fall from grace and it is also the very moment that the atoning blood does not cover your sins. Your sin is now your own. You are by choice emitting low frequencies in the face of HF as if to mock Him and the consequences of your actions will soon be made manifest into your life. God is not mocked. You reap/receive *exactly* what you sow/send out.

If an evil spirit can bring you to a place of 'questioning' God's goodness, God's character, and that which God has revealed to you, what he has gotten you to do is to assert yourself over God to judge God like he, the devil or demon spirit, himself has. Evil spirits love to mock, belittle, and blaspheme God/Truth and their main desire is to draw you into their own way of thinking and behaving and eventually into their realm. It makes them feel powerful and godlike, reaffirming the lies that they love. It is their 'goal' to get you to question and assert yourself over the Truth too, and by that I mean that which you know is right in your heart and they draw you into sin with the forbidden fruit; the promise of your own goodness apart from God.

Look at this scripture again:

7 Submit yourselves therefore to God. Resist the devil, and he will flee from you.
James 4:7 (KJV)

Only two forces are present, God and the devil, not the Devil, but an unclean spirit devil. You fall prey to a devil if you don't submit to God who is the Truth (again by truth I don't mean a theology but what God has revealed to you in the secret of your own closet/heart as to what is right or wrong.) It is in the submitting that the correct or incorrect pathways of your life are taken. Who you submit to will determine who is bringing you the solutions to your life as this will be the frequency you are emitting and receiving. Therefore, it can be concluded that all people are indeed spiritual as all is Spirit. There are just two kinds of spiritual people as there are only two sets of frequencies that can be emitted from your spirit.

8 Draw nigh to God, and he will draw nigh to you. Cleanse *your* hands, *ye* sinners; and purify *your* hearts, *ye* double minded.   James 4:8

If you pull near to the Truth you automatically pull away from the lie, right? Any spirit who speaks contrary to what God has personally shown you in your heart is a spirit that must be resisted. You have to resist low frequency thoughts no matter who or what they come through. This is how God is creating sons and daughters of Truth in the earth; children of High Frequency. Look again at the scripture above. Your hands will be 'clean' if you obey. Whereas a spirit that did not obey would be unclean. Unclean spirits are spirits that move from wrong thinking and their hearts/frequencies are not pure. They bring a double mind to you. In other words, you will be trying to know(follow) good/high frequencies and evil/low frequencies simultaneously. God wants you to know only good because evil will destroy your spirit and lead you to eternal death. God's goal is to save your spirit from death, bring forth a soul that loves the Truth more than lies and save you. These spirits are His children; His sons and daughters. This is His objective concerning you and all your life on earth will be based on this principle/plan that God has pertaining to you. The unclean spirits objective for you is to destroy you and add another soul to their army as they hope to one day take over the throne of heaven and fully know and experience themselves as gods. They come to kill, steal, and destroy God/High Frequencies in you. Little do they know that God is all there really is and if they would have loved the Truth, they would have seen the futility of their actions and their lives would not have been wasted.

Here we see the heart of God and clues as to whose are really His:

7 Then said Jesus unto them again, Verily, verily, I say unto you, I am the door of the sheep.

8 All that ever came before me are thieves and robbers: but the sheep did not hear them.

When you really want the truth, nothing else will do. Your heart cannot be at peace with anyone's version of truth nor is it happy with hypocrisy and religions. Your heart can only welcome His voice/HF and only those who hear His voice will be able to hear your voice if your words are His words. If you are only interested in and seeking high frequency thoughts you will also walk with those who are doing the same thing.

9 I am the door: by me if any man enter in, he shall be saved, and shall go in and out, and find pasture.

The only road to peace, love, and the kingdom of Heaven is by the Living Word— truth alive in your heart. It is by Him that you are saved and able to live and move and get what your soul and spirit needs as He is all. Your spirit is either being nurtured by the Father or by devils at any given moment. Jesus is the door because He is the way. You cannot enter by any other way than how he lived. By giving your life to Him(Him in you) you will begin to emit and receive God's Spirit/Frequencies and find pasture or in other words—what you need to sustain you. This means that you are emitting high frequencies and He Himself is responding to you. He hears you, recognizes you, you are His child and He is fathering your spirit. Jesus is the Way and all who believe that He is the begotten Son of God and who give their lives to His ways are indeed His and He died for their sin/wrong thoughts/low frequencies.

10 The thief cometh not, but for to steal, and to kill, and to destroy: I am come that they might have life, and that they might have *it* more abundantly. Jn 10:7-10 (KJV)

Jesus came so we would have life (high frequencies) and have them more abundantly. This must be our attitude in life towards others and ourselves. We should be seeking to only establish correct emotions, thoughts, and ways in people. If you see yourself taking from others, hurting them, and destroying their hearts just know that this was not God moving in you. These ways belong to the unclean spirits— the thieves.

The thieves rob you of Life itself. These are those other spirits that come to feed you their poison, their lies, their ways, and their love of self. They come to steal God/HF in you. If they can do it, they win and you lose! Can you get them before they get you? If you successfully resist them, they will flee but what if you cannot spot them and you move upon them unwarily? Can you spot them in others? Let me help you. What people in your life come to you only to put you down, steal your love, and trash your soul? Who shows up knocking at your door to use you? How many people do you know that only say hello with a hidden agenda in their back pocket? Unclean spirits are using people to do their work. They want to establish all low frequency type thoughts and emotions in you. They are attacking you from the inside and the outside.

Who seeks to destroy HF in your life? Who is out to reaffirm what is not true in your world? Who builds anger in your heart, mocks you, and puts you down at any given chance? Anyone who tempts you and encourages you into sin is working for devils. Who wants you to complain, slander, gossip, worship them or yourself, be proud, lustful, and to hate and/or be cruel to others? Who is leading you into wrong thoughts and ways; complimenting or deceiving you, lying to you, encouraging you into things that are not right, patting your back and just hoping that you will return the lie to them? Can you see the demon spirit now? He is everywhere and very very busy.

The other 'voices' that try to shepherd you are in you just like the Shepherd. These voices, that seem to be just beyond the hearing for most, encourage you and prod you into many things you later on regret. They are outside of you and inside of you, pulling you into their dark world. This is the voice of this low frequency world. The world that Jesus would not pray for. The evil ones don't come to really feed you but to feed off of you. They will kill your soul, steal what is true in your heart, and destroy you if you believe them and let them.

The Word, the Good Shepherd, is the Truth. He is the good Shepherd because He leads you to Life, to the Truth for your benefit which is exactly how you are to relate to others. All the good that you do in others lives must only be done for their benefit. I want to reiterate the importance of understanding

35

my definition of Truth. I am not talking about the theology of others or yourself as truth...that is not truth. I am talking about what your heart knows because God revealed it to your inner man.

There is little to no love of Truth in the heart of a proud man. He loves himself the most and he is his own truth. All the good that he does is to prove his own goodness, not for the love of what is right.

Thankfully, time is designed to destroy pride, for in time man will see and come to know who he really is as his body ages and fades away before his very eyes and he sees himself diminish in the earth, becoming worm food and a long forgotten memory. Then, for the hard of heart, the grave becomes the final blow to the proud man. What is he then? What does he possess? He watches silently as his things are sold and his body laid in the ground and he is soon forgotten. He gets to see himself as he really is, nothing without God.

Demons and unclean spirits are proud and not interested in pleasing God. They seek to be god and to establish 'another truth' in you. It is what they do and who they are. When you hear these kinds of thoughts in your mind, the kind that pull you away from your inner knowing, know that you are being helped into them by a force that you can't see. The Holy Spirit would never even prompt such a question into your mind as to steal, hurt, or destroy would He? So all evil spirits lie and God does not. God is not human either, remember we 'fell' from our state of perfection. God is a Spirit—the All-

Spirit-God. Our only likeness is that our spirit functions as His does. Once God has shown you the truth on something in your life in a revealing way and you know the Truth in an inspired manner, the first thing that will happen is a liar, namely a devil, will come to steal what has been given to you by the Father. This is God's plan. Your Father wants you to stand up for what is right and be a man unto Truth; a son of God, not a coward. Will you be valiant for the Truth or will you run like a coward back into the dark recesses of the mind.

Let's look at Mark 4:15.....

The sower soweth the word. And these are they by the way side, where the word is sown; but when they have heard, Satan cometh immediately, and taketh away the word that was sown in their hearts.
Mark 4:14-15 (KJV)

The Greek word for Satan used in this verse means accuser and is not speaking of one entity but means 'the devil or accuser'. Please understand that creation is designed this way on purpose. God is in the business of making sons and daughters. He cannot do this if you don't have a choice between good and evil. When the purpose of the unclean spirit is finished, the books of Life are closed, this realm will be gone.
Devils come immediately to steal the truth from

your heart this is the basis and very root of how unclean spirits work. The only way they can have a home in us is if we let them live there by moving and dwelling within their lies. They cannot live in purity and Truth. They can only dwell in a soul that entertains them and any soul that becomes enlightened to Truth they are immediately removed in that area of your spirit man. Being 'filled with the Holy Spirit' is a phrase the church created. It does not mean that demonic spirits have no access to your spirit. Your spirit transmits and can 'receive' the Holy Spirit, not fill up on Him.

As you begin to transmit the Holy Spirit instead of demonic spirits your aura begins to change. You can't hide or change your aura by will. It is glowing like a light bulb and emitting frequencies. Even I can tell your weaknesses by your color. It isn't hard to see or sense what state you are in spiritually from the outside. Please realize that you can't hide sin from God. He really does 'see' you as you are.

Darkness in your soul shows up in your aura as dark colors. You are actually calling unclean spirits to you and your aura tells it all. Your thoughts are emitting the frequencies that are pulling either negative or positive energy into your own life. Sin (wrong thoughts acted on) really does make you sick because it diminished God's life giving presence to your own spirit.

Some people like to believe that 'once saved always saved'. This thinking allows unclean spirits a lot of room to move as the person will not feel the need to ever repent of any low frequency thoughts. Feeling secure in their sin they just stay on course straight to Hades. Just because a person has come to God at some point in their life does not mean that they are saved. Salvation does not work like that. God said that there would be many who were His who would become 'lukewarm' and He would spew them out of His mouth. A lukewarm Christian is a person who takes the truth and mingles it with lies to create the result that appeals to them and they proceed to live from their own imagination. These will be spat out and put away from God's presence and are even more reprehensible to him than the worst sinner. This proves the 'once saved always saved' is false theology. Again, deception comes from love of self. People who love what is wrong in them don't want to truly repent. They want the false confidence that it is okay to live and love sin. They want to believe the lie that as long as you say the magical sinners prayer and pretend you are saved; you are saved. This thought is based on deception and is a low frequency thought. You cannot fool God, okay? So why try?

Every time the Holy Spirit speaks truth unclean spirits immediately speak and argue against Him and they do it 'in your spirit man'. They have access to every human being on earth and can move by merely a thought. Time holds no barrier for them. Where ever they want to go, they simply move by thinking of the place they want to be and they move instantly. This has been proven in exorcisms and

39

your own spirit, even though tethered to a body, can do this to some extent. Psychics also have proven this by calling the dead up in them instantly and communicating via the mind.

No one is exempt from demonic influences. Even Jesus was tempted and He was sinless. Being tempted or propositioned by evil has nothing to do with your holiness or non-holiness. You have the volume control on your radio and the dial select button. Who are you tuning in to and how loud are you wishing to hear them? Unclean spirits have an ability to examine you, speak to you, and tempt you no matter what level of maturity you have in Christ. This world is designed that way. It is your responsibility to tune them out. You cannot do this if you are caught up in their voices and think they are you.

14 The sower soweth the word.

The Holy Spirit is the Sower and He is placing the seed of Truth into your heart 24/7. He is faithful and wishes all to come to the Truth. He tells all of that which is right and that which is not right. All who are goodhearted will hear him and bring forth fruit. He's the still quiet voice in you that always makes you feel ashamed for having done something wrong. Even the littlest things are brought to attention in Him. Did you take the biggest piece of pie? Your conscious will let you know the truth right down to the way you drive! God is with you always and people hate it! They try to make God shut up and He won't. He loves His creation and if you go to eternal hell, it will be your own fault for doing such as you will have had to give it a great deal of effort.

15 And these are they by the way side, where the word is sown; but when they have heard, Satan cometh immediately, and taketh away the word that was sown in their hearts.

Mark 4:14-15 (KJV)

Again, the word Satan in Greek means the devil or demon. Satan is not omnipresent and cannot be in the heart of everyone everywhere around the world at once so it cannot be speaking of him directly but indirectly as a 'way' of thinking/low frequency. This isn't just one entity going around attacking one person at a time afflicting them and leading them astray. Wouldn't it be nice if it were?! The devil is that voice that says, "its okay to be rude, they were rude too. The biggest piece of pie is rightfully yours cause you got there first," these lies wouldn't work if you didn't like being rude or love pie.

The energy behind all lies and deception come from devils or demons. The father of them is Satan who isn't a human being or an unclean spirit himself, but Lucifer, the Leviathon. Every time God hands you the Truth in your heart a devil comes to steal it away—every single time! Satan is not omnipresent and the devil or unclean spirit is

41

present with and around us all the time. Paul lets us know that they move through the air and are like air. The air is present with you but you cannot see it yet it is an integral part of your life. You breath it, it enters into you and leaves you.

2 Wherein in time past ye walked according to the course of this world, according to the prince of the power of the air, the spirit that now worketh in the children of disobedience:

Eph 2:1-2 (KJV)

Devils have a 'course' or a 'way' that they move. When you didn't know truth or have high frequency thoughts to move from, you moved from this other way. Jesus came to show you the correct way; the correct frequency. He died for all your wrong thoughts/LF. The prince of the power of the air is the same as the spirit that now works in the children of disobedience. It is the unclean spirit that enter and works in children who disobey God/Truth. They may be working on getting obedient ones to fall but they can only work in and use the disobedient, these are the ones who follow them and think their thoughts, speak their words, and carry out their actions in the earth. They persecute the ones who won't obey their LF until they give in.

Among whom also we all had our conversation in times past in the lusts of our flesh, fulfilling the

42

desires of the flesh and of the mind; and were by nature the children of wrath, even as others.

Eph 2:3 (KJV)

Among these unclean spirits we all (that's everyone) had our conversation in times past because we were moving in and from the lusts of our flesh. We all spoke and emitted low frequencies. We were fulfilling the desires of our 'minds' and were by nature the children of anger. This nature will begin to change the moment you give your life to God and it must change in order for us to be saved. We must die daily. Out with the old frequency/man and in with the new. Your heart will be angry when you move from low frequency thoughts because of its immediate opposition to God who is Peace.

How can you change the nature of a man? This is what the Holy Spirit will do in your life, if you give your life to Him. If we don't listen to the truth revealed to us, we are not the good ground. We will not produce the fruit of truth in our lives. God usually speaks to you through a wordless knowing. It is a feeling or understanding that you will encounter in you. The moment you turn from the correct feeling or thought the negative LF voices begin to speak up and overwhelm you. Then you take up your argument with the voices against His Truth in you and become the enemy of God, sympathizing with yourself, you drown in self pity.

Your heart gets angry as it lives in condemnation, and you get lost in the devils thoughts and emotions. You at once begin excusing, blaming, and resenting yourself and others and no matter what you do, you can't make the bad feeling go away for moving against the inner knowing that you had in the beginning. These voices that torment and argue are the flesh that Paul spoke of and are LF voices within you. Those who try to say that our flesh has nothing to do with unclean spirits would be wise to reread Eph. 2:3 until your eyes open up. Matter is nothing but spirit manifest. Your matter becomes the thoughts you entertain. Who are you having your conversation amongst? It never says that we are having our conversations with ourselves as many preach. This is irrefutable proof that Paul was talking about demonic activity in people. Remember, Satan is not omnipresent.

7 And the LORD said unto Satan, Whence comest thou? Then Satan answered the LORD, and said, From going to and fro in the earth, and from walking up and down in it.

Job 1:7 (KJV)

Satan can only be in one place at a time. He was sitting in the tree talking to Eve, he walks to and fro throughout the earth, one day he will be cast into the eternal lake of fire. He is not omnipresent picking on anyone and everyone on earth simultaneously. So who is this 'devil' that we must resist if it isn't

44

Satan? It is the unclean spirit that Jesus cast out of people and many were healed as a result of doing such.

Who has taught the church that Satan is against each one of us and there in person? When is the last time anyone has actually bumped into him? Who is at this very moment concealing the truth about unclean spirits? Why does the church hold on to the doctrine that Satan is omnipresent? Who are they teaching people to fear and why? Why do they preach that Nephilims are unclean spirits when it is NOT in the bible?

If Satan isn't running around in people then where is he really at? Just what is he doing in the earth right now?

2 And he laid hold on the dragon, that old serpent, which is the Devil, and Satan, and bound him a thousand years,

3 And cast him into the bottomless pit, and shut him up, and set a seal upon him, that he should deceive the nations no more, till the thousand years should be fulfilled: and after that he must be loosed a little season.

Rev 20:2-3 (KJV)

Satan may not be at your back door talking to you, but he is not unable to affect people right now. He is not 'inoperative' but appears to have restrictions which has kept him from our dimension. I personally believe that that was part of the victory of the cross. According to scripture Satan is at work deceiving the nations. That is what the bible says he is doing at this very moment and that he is free enough to have to be bound in order to separate him from those living through the thousand year reign. I believe that he is stuck in a very low frequency and cannot rise.

How he is able to influence the world I'm sure is crafty and quite impressive to our limited mentality. He is an age old creature after all who once was adorned in wisdom and beauty. The beast and the new one world government will be by his design and the death of many Christians in the world will be at his hand and allowed by God to refine His own children. Again, Satan is the deceiver and the ultimately deceived. He thinks he's building his kingdom, destroying God, and becoming God; meanwhile Satan will merely help refine God's children. Satan will formulate a number for all mankind and seek to root out of the earth all those who are truly the Father's children and destroy them so that the earth will be his. He believes he is destroying God's children, meanwhile he is actually helping develop and create them. His plans will not remain as he is LF. His ways are not upheld by the Father. All who move from LF thoughts and ways are doing dead works. Their works will not remain in the earth. So if you move from lust, greed, pride, or those kinds of things what you have done will one day be destroyed by the Fire of Truth along with all other LF's thoughts and ways. So we see that Satan is not inoperative but fully doing that which he was created to do in so much that he will be able to wage war against the hosts of heaven soon.

Who are Satan's enemies? It is not the religious minded as they do and live for themselves, like Satan. Satan has always warred against the Truth. Since the beginning of our time there has been the war of good and evil, Truth and lies. Those who love the Truth are the enemies of Satan. Just as it was in the days of Jesus. The Pharisees or religious ones were the one's who did most of Satan's work and the ones who killed the Truth, nailing Him to their own cross/ambition. This is how the Truth dies in you. You kill Him for your own ambitions. Satan's helpers and enemies are the same today as they have been since creation began—he hates the Truth/God. Hence, only those who love the Truth are his enemies. Satan is very religious and knows the bible inside out, quoting scripture fluently and effortlessly as he did to Jesus. He is the father of lies and loves twisting the truth to destroy the works of God's hand. All those who love and obey the Truth are Satan's enemies and all demons/unclean spirits come to destroy the Truth in you. They come to steal from you, kill you, and destroy you; spirit, soul, and body. They can only do this if they can remove the truth from your heart. This is what they want.

47

The only way to defeat a lie is with the truth, right? There is no middle ground. That which is.... is. It needs no one to substantiate it. This is God...He simply is. Everything is either right or wrong, is it not? You are on one side or the other in what you think and do. All attempts to ride a middle ground and claim your own religion and ways aside from His will meet full disaster and are still lies. For everything outside of Him is lies and will come to nothing.

Enter ye in at the strait gate: for wide *is* the gate, and broad *is* the way, that leadeth to destruction, and many there be which go in thereat:

Because strait *is* the gate, and narrow *is* the way, which leadeth unto life, and few there be that find it.

Matt 7:13-14 (KJV)

The wisdom here is shown. There are many paths to lies because there are many liars to listen too. Many will go down these paths trying to find a way to fulfill their own lusts. They will seek to enter heaven but cannot because they don't really love the Truth/God. They love themselves and even their religion is based upon self adoration and preservation. Spiritual gifts are just for the bragging, hours of bible studying to show themselves wise and win in debates, fasting is done only to prove how 'spiritually devoted' they are, boasting, diplomas, titles, and monetary gain; all is vanity. All those who do these things are heading through that

48

wide gate which leads to complete destruction. There is no difference between a Christian who uses God for self gain than a Pharisee who used God for self gain. Jesus called their father the devil because they moved from evil spirits and evil motives for self gain.

The narrow Truth is often very hard to hear. People generally hate the truth, especially about themselves. Pride cannot bear to see itself for what it is— a lie. However, if one is willing to see the Truth then one will find that narrow pathway to eternal life. Will you leave yourself behind? Are you willing to nail self (belief in an existence outside of God) to the cross, consider yourself dead to this world and its ways and live for Him? Will you seek the truth, to know how it really is, no matter what it costs you personally? Do you realize that you really are dead without the Truth to redeem you anyway? All people need to do is see the Truth of their own existence and they will find salvation.

These principals are the very basis of the bible itself. All who love Truth— love God, for God is Truth. He is Reality. When honesty hurts, be it known that lies have a home in your heart and honesty is only painful to a person when that person doesn't want to see the Truth. If one could but realize that without Honesty and Truth present there is no defense against unclean spirits nor will you find salvation.

All who move from the Holy Spirit are God's.

They love the Truth which sets them apart from the world and world's ways. The opposite is also true. All who love lies are of Satan. In essence, Satan moves in every lie lover in the world. Although he is not directly present, in spirit he is because these are his children who do as he does; they emit low frequencies in order to overcome and destroy you. It is as if he is present around the world because they carry out his wishes, his thoughts, and his ways—the frequencies he moves in.

Who do you promote in your life? Who's message are you preaching? Who are you honoring? What are you emitting? If you are moving and doing everything for self gain, trying to prove how amazing and wonderful you are, in love with your self, and living for you.....how can you be a child of Truth? You are either a person of principle or the principal person.

We all have a certain amount of deception in us and that is the same thing as saying that we all have some measure of demonic influence in our lives. However, it isn't like the movies make demonic possession out to be, nor am I suggesting that you are completely possessed. The movies paint a sordid picture..... you know what I mean, heads turning full circle, dolls talking, and walls bleeding. This is actually another ploy from demonic spirits to remain hidden. They teach the world that this is what demonic possession looks like and it isn't true in 99.9 percent of the cases.

I'm not saying that those things don't happen on occasion either, what I am saying is that if you don't resist the devil he won't flee. He's already there. He is waiting to see what you will do and if you don't resist him he'll just set up camp. From his comfy camp he proceeds to steal the truth from your heart. If allowed to grow, he'll destroy your soul, kill you, and destroying your life. If this sounds like your life, know that this is the flashing neon sign that you didn't successfully resist him. Soon, he'll oust you right out of your own body and move on to his next victim. Every demonic spirit brings death to you because they move in the low frequency range which cuts God's life giving energy from your own spirit and body.

Everyone's got their demons. Everyone argues with those voices in their heads. Little wicked whispers that we often would die of embarrassment if anyone were to witness or over hear them. Horrible dark sides that we feel alive in us and we all have them because we all live in a low frequency realm. These are the voices that whisper wicked thoughts into your ears and cause you to give into their evil schemes. I'm talking about what most Christians calmly term as your flesh which is also accepted as 'okay' nowadays and completely overlooked as long as you raise your hands in worship and toss in your dollars on the offering plate and bump up to the alter for a stale cracker and a squirt of juice and scream 'grace'.

This 'flesh' is Satan with us. These voices belong to the realm of darkness, death, and corruption, not to God and this is the 'devil' that comes to destroy you should you not resist. Can you be humble enough to admit that devils are present? Look again at this verse in James:

Draw nigh to God, and he will draw nigh to you. Cleanse *your* hands, *ye* sinners; and purify *your* hearts, *ye* double minded.

James 4:8 (KJV)

A wicked heart is one that moves on and from demonic thoughts/frequencies. It is when we pull away from God's thoughts/high frequencies that devils draw near to us. The battlefield is in your mind/heart. A wicked heart is a wicked soul and it is with the heart that man believes unto salvation because he is believing the Truth. It is also with his heart that he believes unto death. Believing lies will kill you.

10 For with the heart man believeth unto righteousness; and with the mouth confession is made unto salvation.

Romans 10:10 (KJV)

When you deal with unclean spirits, whether you are exorcising them or they are tempting you, you must realize that they only use the truth to sell their lies. Lying is what they love to do. Their father taught them well and he is very proud of his children. You must not rely solely upon an unclean spirit's word for anything. They will say and do whatever they can to avoid any harm to themselves and often even protect their host for personal reasons, considering them their own. This spirit may also sometimes be referred to as a spirit guide and some falsely think they are angels. They are spirits that are using people and consider them their own. Unclean spirits really do view people as their own property. It is where they live and function and if an unclean spirit lives within a person from childhood they really lay claim to that soul and spirit as their own, viewing them much like we do a house or a home even though their very presence eventually brings death to their host and even your children are often viewed by them as theirs. Sometimes they name children and people don't even realize it. I've seen it happen. I know these are hard facts to hear, but the Truth is the Truth. These spirits are reliving their lives through people and people generally do not realize what is going on.

Necromancy, which means communication with the dead, was prohibited by God because the most sure way to get lost is to follow the lost. When people seek the advice and wisdom of the dead they will end up there themselves. God does not wish anyone to perish. This is why death was the penalty for seeking the friendship and fellowship of the dead. Every person who does not take God's advice and counsel is getting their advice and wisdom from another source....this source is from the unclean spirit. This is why you are to avoid deep nurturing type friendships with anyone who is not submissive to God and moving from a substantial amount of correct thoughts and ways. Don't be fooled by their claiming that they want to follow God and just can't seem to find Him, but look at the fruits in their lives. Do they love and practice sin? If so, stay away from them. One who dwells in the Light cannot have peaceful relationship with a person who loves the dark. There is nothing personal about it, just simple facts, folks. Be wise and Wisdom will keep you.

God never withholds His wisdom and guidance from anyone who seriously seeks it. If a person claims they really want to find the Truth, but just can't quite ever come up with it in their lives this is a warning sign that they are liars and love lies. God promises to never hide the truth from anyone who asks. Therefore, they are lying to your face. To hang out with them will most likely draw darkness into your own soul, so be careful and wise with whom you congregate and how you fellowship. David said it best.

4 A froward heart shall depart from me: I will not know a wicked *person*.

Psalms 101:3-4 (KJV)

You can feel what another person is emitting. When someone gives you the creeps it means that that person was emitting a frequency far different from yours. If you can sense what a person is emitting, how easy is it for someone who is pure energy; in other words, a spirit without a body to do the same?

Avoid people who love wrong ways and thoughts. They will try to drag you into their sin and wrong way of living and lead you astray. Be wise, *you become your friends.*

Learn to protect the Truth in you as a most prized possession, more valuable than rubies or diamonds and never cast what is precious in you before a demonic spirit in another. Don't trust your heart/jewel to a thief or your heart will be robbed as that person takes your precious revelations and things from heaven and uses them to hurt and destroy you; doing the work of devils.

Remember, devils are after God in you, the Truth in your heart, with all their might. This is what they want; what they must have to get your soul. They do it anyway they can and use other people to destroy the good in your heart. War and fight the good fight of faith, be wise and don't open your heart up to devil's opinions and friendships that come from hell. If you see a person whose flesh is in control of them, such as a person who cannot stop gossiping, slandering, hating, resenting, being jealous, and cannot control their mouth, do not fellowship with them. You don't have to be rude or cruel, just avoid them as Paul suggests. If you must respond to them, do so in a firm kind way hoping that they will get better, making sure that your only words are words that help them and seek nothing for yourself. This will keep your actions pure. The moment you make any situation about you, is the moment you will fall into sin. If you cannot speak in an unselfish manner do not say a word. This will bring less sin upon everyone involved. Just hold your peace and walk away. Only speak when you see it is wise.

Don't battle foolishly and hand the enemy your heart. Our battle, the real battle, is not directly against this world, people, or the manifestations of spirits through people, but against deceit in our own hearts. God doesn't want us to speak, follow, and take advice from the dead. They have missed the mark, lost the battle, and failed. He doesn't want you to follow in their footsteps which is also why you are to avoid people who follow the dead in them; this also is necromancy.

Now, why would it be a crime to speak with the dead if they were not really the dead and are not present? Many theologians argue that other spirits that are evil are pretending to be the dead yet God clearly stated that we aren't to speak with the dead. Is God lying to us? His scripture tells us that they are the dead and that we are not to speak with them or make sacrifices to them. So where is this false doctrine coming from? Who told the theologians to lie to us about the dead? Who wanted us to not know that the dead were not killing us? With this kind of misinformation exorcisms are not done properly and demons are overlooked and allowed entrance, access, and dominion over people. How convenient for the unclean spirit, don't you think? Another reason people deny the origin of unclean spirits is because they are afraid that if a demon speaks and they respond that they have committed the sin of necromancy. This is another ploy by the demonic spirit to stay in control of people. After all, since you cannot speak with the dead you cannot cast them out either, again...how convenient—for the unclean spirit that is. Unclean spirits are far sharper than people give them credit for they are seeing both worlds at the same time whereas we are privy to seeing very little of theirs. God never said not to speak with the dead, he said not to 'follow' the dead. Jesus spoke with the dead and he was sinless. Right there is proof of a serious false doctrine taught by demonic spirits within the church. God is not the author of this teaching then is He?

How dangerous is it to teach people that their enemy cannot reach them and that they are not to engage the enemy should they actually bump into him and that he isn't who he is? Who gains in those scenarios? These are just more lies spoken by the demonic realm and brought forth in their religious leaders and theologians to hide the Truth from real believers. Unclean spirits are exactly what the bible says they are. They are 'unclean spirits' which have not been cleansed by the Spirit of Truth. They passed from this life only to find themselves in a dry place— a place of 'dust'. They are living in the place where man's flesh was brought forth from but without a body they feel no warmth and their spirits have no place to rest or abode. Ghosts emit low frequencies. You can buy the meters from many retailers. It is commonly known.

Look at the following verse closely. God said I am the living and you are seeking the 'dead'. He didn't say, "you are seeking Satan or Nephilims". He said that those who sought counsel with familiar spirits were taking counsel with the dead. Familiar spirits 'are' the souls of the dead. This is what God Himself said yet people teach and preach otherwise, claiming it is of God. Is God lying? He cannot.

And when they shall say unto you, Seek unto them that have familiar spirits, and unto wizards that peep, and that mutter: should not a people seek unto their God? for the living to the dead?
Isaiah 8:19 (KJV)

Now, what spirit would desire for the church to believe that familiar spirits are NOT the spirits of the dead? What spirit would try and hide itself to protect itself from being found out?

Familiar spirits are termed 'familiar' because they are familiar with and to you. Almost all demonic possessions and oppressions are from unsaved deceased relatives. The word familiar is used for a reason. The translation of this word is very informative. The word used is 'ob' and it represents the idea of prattling a father's name. Unclean spirits usually stay within the family on the father's side. The word that God used to describe the spirits of the dead that were being channeled is quite accurate and has nothing to do with Nephilims.

Wizards and those that 'have' a devil or an unclean spirit would 'peep'. The word 'peep' in Hebrew means to chatter or whisper. In effect, God was saying that those who speak for the dead should be stoned. The 'dead' or souls of the unsaved are unclean. It was common knowledge in Jesus' day and nothing has changed to this day except that the Church doesn't know or want to know who they are and refuse to see the truth. They love their false theology on heaven and hell as it is instrumental in their brainwashing process.

Another reason that people have not seen the light is because it is an uncomfortable thing to know. However, if they could actually grab a hold of the truth on this issue, unclean spirits would be in huge trouble. Many, many people would get healed and delivered. As it is, unclean spirits hide and destroy us from the inside out stealthily in a premeditated manner. They go about reinforcing all the beliefs, illness, and emotions that kept them from entering heaven and kill the souls and bodies of their hosts. Every lie(low frequency) is backed by them, encouraged, grown, and reinforced. Will the church ever come into the knowledge of the origin and activities of the unclean spirit? Be wise and seek the Truth no matter the personal cost. One day soon it will be too late to do so.

Three

The Dybbuk

and other evidentiary findings......

What was the understanding of demonic spirits when Jesus walked on planet earth? Was there a controversy amongst the religious community? When Jesus roamed the dusty streets of Jerusalem there was no mystery concerning the origin of unclean spirits. Everyone knew. It was written in the bible scrolls that the disciples had and was common knowledge. The Jews called them the 'dybbuk'. Get your dictionary out and look for yourself. Here is what mine says.....

Dybbuk: a demon, or the soul of a dead person, that enters the body of a living person and directs the person's conduct, exorcism being possible only by a religious ceremony.-Webster

Do you think it is just coincidental that the Jews knew exactly who demons were? The disciples knew full well that unclean spirits were the souls of the dead and it is still common knowledge amongst the oldest cultures in the world.

61

In Japan and other cultures a fine meal is set out for the dead or an offering of some kind and the dead show up and ring a bell to let the living know that they are pleased with the offering.

In Chinese culture in Singapore whoever is closest to the dead body or had spent the most time around the dead person is considered the least clean and therefore they can legally obtain most of the dead person's possessions. They may not even realize the reason for their own belief. The spirit of that dead person would most likely enter the person who was nearest it upon death and so the dead are allowed to live on with their possessions as they live on in them.

I can understand why people run from the truth about unclean spirits. It is very uncomfortable to know that your loved one didn't make it and has become a foe. Especially if your faith is like theirs! I also understand why it is not a well known fact. It is a most unpleasant thing to know. Please realize that God is still working with them and they will be brought forward in the second judgment. We are to distance ourselves from the dead. If people knew their dead loved ones were present, what would they do? History tends to repeat itself and in the East they worship their dead. How many people would decide that God was Love and that he would want them to help their dead relatives and soul mates? How many people would follow and converse with the dead knowingly and lovingly? I am sure there would be many. History always repeats itself and in the Eastern cultures they do knowingly and lovingly follow the dead; building shrines unto their ancestors. I hope that you do not be so foolish as to repeat the mistake of conversing with the dead.

Demonic spirits have a function. They are part of the design of the earth and although God does not wish any to perish, all who turn from Truth find themselves in the company of one another. This is why sin leads to death, the realm of the dead. I have pondered a lot upon the wisdom behind combining the two worlds and I see that without a choice and a power pulling us away from Truth we would not be creatures of free will nor would we have an environment that causes us to grow spiritually. So in a sort of bizarre way they are doing His work. They are helping create sons and daughters of heaven by creating the situations that help us grow. After all, how can one learn to forgive if a trespass is never to occur?

I know that we are not suppose to live in a way that entertains unclean spirits and I know that Jesus commanded us to cast them out of people; showing His view of their actions. If unclean spirits take up residency in you, you will likely die of the same illness that they had when they died. This is also not the will of the Father and He gave us explicit right to cast them out. We are to heal the sick, raise the dead, and cast out unclean spirits. They are not our friends in that we should just live with them, sympathize with or for them, and let them destroy us or others and feel some sort of heroic emotion as if we are helping their cause. God let me know that any sympathy for them is not pleasing to Him. Are we more holy than He that we should put our views of their fate and situation ahead of what He has done? We walk on dangerous ground anytime we try to out 'holy' the Father.

I hope to try some methods of exorcisms out on the heavily possessed in the near future. I am curious to see if they will work but I believe that I have found much wisdom in the way that Muslims do their exorcisms and I will discuss their methods in greater detail in the near future. Basically, the Muslim believe that demons are a creature unto themselves and they call them djinn. They believe that the djinn reproduce. This is because they have found families in the realm of the dead and people of all ages. I've been reading and pondering their beliefs and because I have the understanding of who unclean spirits really are, all their pieces are beginning to make sense when viewed with the Truth. The djinn are clearly the souls of the dead and often in the videos I have seen them give human names and tell how long they have been in the person upon death, why they are in them, and how they died.

Being without a body must be torture in that realm. The bible describes it as a dry and and restless place. I cannot imagine the horror of it and people that realize that it is true usually cannot bear it and pretend that I am wrong, struggling to forget what was revealed to their inner man. In full denial, they proceed to despise you as you remind them of their sin for having turned a deaf ear to the truth. It is a hard truth to bear. What loved one is living in or around you? Who lost their way in your family and is trying to live their lives in you? It is a very tough thing to face and I really do understand why people choose to not see it and to see their loved ones somewhere sleeping or in heaven playing and having fun in some happy hunting ground. Unfortunately this is costing people their own lives prematurely and also in many many cases it is costing souls as well. Demons are able to destroy the living because the living refuse to see the truth about the dead.

If you are wondering who is living in and through your life you may already know. Many people make comments like, "you are just like your grandma" and "there's a little bit of your Ma or Pa in you". Plus, look at your dreams. Reoccurring dead relatives is also a sign of who is moving in you. I can tell you how to see the dead on your own face but in my experience this also brings the demonic spirit forwards and so I will decline for now. Some people are too possessed to do this and one person I know was overtaken by the demon as it arose.

Please use wisdom when dealing with spirits. If they could kill you instantly, I assure you, they would. So have faith in the fact that God has assigned you angel(s) to watch over you and that you are not your own. Demonic spirits have no wisdom that you need to know. There is no reason to drill them or get their expertise on anything. Wisdom belongs to God, not demons. Therefore, do not be foolish and seek the communication with the dead. God is not pleased with it. If you have a question, His Spirit is there to answer it. I've yet to see good results from calling on an unclean spirit to get an answer on an issue in anyone's life and God was wise when he commanded people to not follow and fellowship with the lost.

Do you realize that those who are demon possessed on earth are in essence the living dead? To fellowship, take guidance, and cherish the friendships of this world is to turn your back on God. It is a serious thing to commune and fellowship lovingly with sinners/wrong thinkers in their sin/wrong thinking. Think about this the next time someone comes to you for sympathy. Sympathy belongs to God. You are to feel for Him, not for people who want to hang on to their egos. God does not wish that any should perish. He wants all to come to salvation. You simply cannot find the path of Life speaking to the dead. If they had wisdom they wouldn't be where they are at.

I came across a poll recently that said that over 50 percent of people have seen a ghost or in other words.... an unclean spirit. People are very aware unconsciously that spirits are present and that the dead can communicate with the living. Many people practice communication for a living. How many illnesses could be simply removed by casting the demon out and closing the doors? How many thousands of people have died needlessly? How many have we put on drugs, fried their brains, or locked away? Too many.......may God give us wisdom to overcome. Poor leadership will cause entire races to become extinct.

A true leader will always lead people back to the Truth in themselves. They will never seek to fulfill themselves at or on the expense of another person. They will seek to hook you up with God, not themselves. They know that you must have guidance from the Holy Spirit within you and they know that without that guidance system in place you will perish. Their concern is for your true well being, for your soul, not their own fake image, glory, and ego or any such selfish thing like fame or money. Therefore I speak the Truth to you knowing it will make me less popular and if I wanted to build a huge ministry this would be the worst thing I could do. I do it because it is the right thing to do, the best thing for your soul, and not because it will make me successful in this world. The only way you can overcome the devil is by submitting to God's presence in you.

Church, as it is designed today, will kill your soul. Systematized religion is of the devil. Get out and find God(the way things really are) in you before you seek to share Him in fellowship in any way with others. How can you bless others if you yourself are lost? If you need help leaving a church ask God, He will help you. He doesn't want you to be a Pharisee; a person guided externally by other spirits.

The dead are in and around us all the time, coming and going. They are the principalities of the air that Paul spoke of. They come and go from people on a consistent basis. If they could just overtake you, you would be dead already. So don't fear, panic, or run......God is not dead. His angels are watching you 24/7.

All things are made by Him. He is in control and this world moves by His spiritual principles. You are confused because His mind is not revealed to yours yet. Sin has a price, that's all. Instead of punching ghosts, one would be far better off to punch sin. If you really want to be free from demonic spirits one must quit sinning. *Sin is the open door.* In order to quit sinning (moving from wrong places in your heart, mind, and soul) you need to have God show you the correct thought, feeling, and understanding and you will easily and effortlessly be able to stop sinning.

Most cases of demonic possession are self inflicted; caused by a sin because one is tuning in to the demon's own frequency in great strength. If the person isn't deathly ill and has time it is better to separate them from the sin(s) that is allowing the unclean spirit entry. This is done through repentance. If you move from a mindset that you can just bust spooks and keep them at bay you will die in your pride. No one can win that fight. You are emitting low frequencies by moving on pride and the demons are coming faster than you can kick them out. I don't believe it can even be done. *The only way to true freedom from demonic spirits is through knowing God in you instead of the demons in you.* The Truth really will set you free. You must seek the Healer first and all else will be added to you. However, this is not possible with the severely possessed and it is those that I would love to see set free. I believe that these were the ones that we were commissioned by Christ to free. I pray that the Lord will show me the most effective way to help others and to permanently remove demonic spirits in the tough cases. I realize that it is entirely possible to close down asylums by releasing all their patients and I hope to be able to bless many by doing such.

Another desire that I have is that I would like to create an environment that draws a person to repentance while simultaneously offering deliverance and anointed teachings and hands on meditation practice. This would minister to a person spirit, soul, and body and heal them in whole and not part. This would be accomplished through simple prayer cabins, seminars, and deliverances for those who need a kick start on their walk with God. I would love to see this environment offered on a global scale.

Throwing demons out is not the complete answer by any means as they most often come right back the next day and the person can end up in a bigger mess then when they began fighting. I have had exorcisms done on myself and I know what I'm talking about. Alone exorcisms simply don't work.

One must know the Truth in their own heart and then freedom comes. Freedom does not come through exorcisms alone. No where in the bible does it say that exorcisms are the answer to mankind's dilemma.

32 And ye shall know the truth, and the truth shall make you free.   John 8:32 (KJV)

Knowing lies in you brings bondage and sickness. Knowing Truth in you brings healing and wellness. God is Truth itself. All that is, is Him. He is pure Science/Mind/Wisdom. There is nothing outside of Him. Demonic spirits work only in the places of disobedience in one's life. It would be ideal for the carnal man if we could just cast out a demon, blame a demon, and go on in sin but it doesn't work that way. The dream is appealing to the flesh, but Reality would have something different to say about that....therefore choose to know Reality and live.

Our wrong thinking is emanating from wrong desires and when we are fulfilling the desires of demons we move towards their realm. This is why they can live in and through us and we think that they are us because we have joined ourselves to them. We invite them in and we move upon them; their thoughts and emotions, and become their children. Just who is possessing who?

4 But God, who is rich in mercy, for his great love wherewith he loved us, 5 Even when we were dead in sins, hath quickened us together with Christ, (by grace ye are saved;) 6 And hath raised *us* up together, and made *us* sit together in heavenly *places* in Christ Jesus:

Just listen to the heart of God. His *great* love and His rich mercy has quickened us, brought us to life to love the Truth. So that we can sit with Christ in heavenly places/HF, not in the places of demonic spirits, in LF. In the places in your heart where hate, anger, malice, self righteousness, and pride once flourished God's Light revealed the truth and showed us what real Love was and in His Light we see Light. He raises your frequencies up so you can hear Him. All who are His are Spirit led, are they not?

7 That in the ages to come he might shew the exceeding riches of his grace in *his* kindness toward us through Christ Jesus.

8 For by grace are ye saved through faith; and that not of yourselves: *it is* the gift of God:

9 Not of works, lest any man should boast.

10 For we are his workmanship, created in Christ Jesus unto good works, which God hath

before ordained that we should walk in them.
Eph 2:1-10 (KJV)

We need to remember that we are His
workmanship and are suppose to be doing good
works, His works. Your salvation cannot come from
your pride. You cannot move from an attitude that
you are saving yourself. It is impossible. This alone
is an evil work. Your salvation is of the Lord. Only
because God decided to have mercy on you, show
you the way, give you the strength to follow it, and
then lead you home can you be saved. Salvation is a
gift. No person has ever been good enough to
deserve it. We have been preordained (enacted by
God's own Mind before we were created) to walk in
His thoughts and ways. Think of it like this....God
turned up His volume so you can hear Him.

Let no man glory in that he has done anything
good of himself. Only God is good and all the good
that is ever wrought forth by our hands came from
His Spirit within us. His Spirit is a gift. Life comes
to us by the grace that He has shown us. We find
Him because He chooses to show us not because we
are super smart and good.

He chose to send Jesus Christ to show us the way
to salvation and to save us through the blood of His
only begotten Son that all who believed into
Him(into his love, his way of life, his heart, his
mind) these will find the Truth and walk in it. For
whatever you are in to comes in to you. All who
come to that cross in humility and sincerity will find

72

salvation. All who come to it for selfish reasons, seeking to know themselves as amazing, wonderful, and spiritually above others will only know themselves in His name and are not His children.

God ordained that we should walk in good works, gave us His salvation, His guiding light, as a gift, and we are to live unto Him for all eternity. It is sobering to know that many will die and forever be lost. God wants everyone to be saved but He also wants you to make your own decision in the matter. Would you want friends who hated you? Neither does He. Therefore, you will have time to see everything before the end of the world. The good news, that one doesn't have to die for their sins, will be told to every person everywhere in every dimension. Will they choose life? No one's demise will be by the hand of God. He is just in all that He does.

The dead are those who have moved to lower vibrations, leaving their bodies behind in most cases. There is still a chance to ascend to HF as the final judgment has not been made by God. The dead missed the Truth at the end of their life however so why would anyone want to communicate and follow the dead? To an honest heart, it makes no sense. What can the dead offer the living? Still, many people try to communicate with the dead. The thumb piano in Africa is an instrument that is used to call the dead. It creates low frequency standing waves that call demonic spirits and helps them to manifest. Some frequency waves deter spirits. These are high ones like those of the shofar horn.

Some people also believe that cities create standing waves which would attract ghosts/unclean spirits. If this were true, it would help escalate the crimes in these areas. A standing wave is a frequency wave that gets trapped inside a building or area causing the sound wave to fall or crash in on itself. It appears that once it reaches and certain intensity it seems to make demonic spirits come full manifest.

(Thumb Piano)

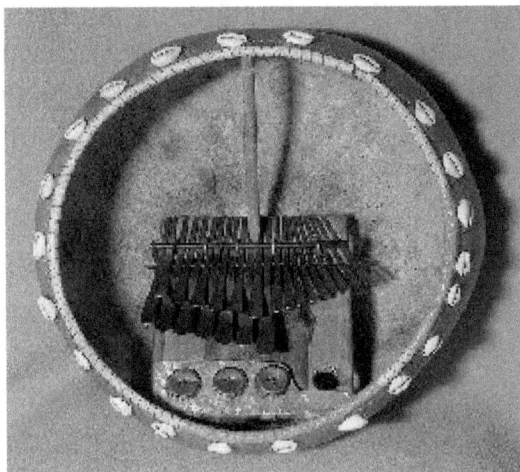

In many countries people fear the demon spirit and sacrifice to appease them. They do not know how to deal with them and don't realize why the demonic spirit is able to enter or how to keep them out. They make deals with them to stay alive. This is not wise and will not work. You will be enslaved to a spirit that despises you and they will run and ruin your life. Never make deals with demons.

You cannot destroy the effects that demons have on your life if you are joined to them. There must be a separation. This can only be done through and by true repentance and God's angels enforcing His spiritual laws. A demons stronghold is sin/wrong thinking and beliefs that you have. Everyone has some. We simply cannot help it. When a person moves from these ways and thoughts that are not of God, demonic spirits get a foothold in one's soul. You cannot begin a fearful barrage of demonic evictions and become well. You cannot move from a spirit of pride, fear, and hate and do the work of God. To save your life the first thing you need to do is abandon it. Trust me, if the demons could instantly kill you you'd be dead already so don't do anything from fear. Fear is a low frequency emotion. All you will do is open up the door to more demons while you are trying to boot out the one's attacking you. You have no power of your own and without God moving through you you are already the demon's toy. Abandon your life on earth. Give it to the One who knows what to do with it. See the truth of your existence, quit playing imaginary games, and begin repenting.

Sickness comes from your faults. I know that is hard to hear but remember what Paul spoke of concerning communion? If we would examine ourselves every time we ate we wouldn't be so sick, so faulty. Communion, as the believers knew it, was a meal and this meal represented them partaking of the sinless nature of Christ in order to destroy their faults.

28 But let a man examine himself, and so let him eat of *that* bread, and drink of *that* cup.

The only way you can partake of Jesus' sinless nature, the nature that has not ONE wrong thought or way in it), is to repent from the wrong thoughts that God shows you. We must examine ourselves and repent. Where are your faults at? If you don't know, how are you going to repent? Exactly how do you plan to come into the fullness of the stature of Christ with your false doctrines and your sin?

29 For he that eateth and drinketh unworthily, eateth and drinketh damnation to himself, not discerning the Lord's body.

Because people refuse to repent and do not discern Him and know Him in them, they are dying in their sins. Sickness comes from sin.

30 For this cause many *are* weak and sickly among you, and many sleep.

Correction of faults brings healing. Why? Demons live within our faults and they make us sick. It is really that simple. Imagine if you actually hated and hunted your faults!

31 For if we would judge ourselves, we should not be judged.

Sickness is our judgment for refusing to see the Truth. This punishment comes to those who call themselves Christians. Paul said it did and he's right. You got back what you sent out. Because we refused to judge rightly within us His judgment is passed upon us in the form of His Spiritual Law. If we would admit the truth and humble ourselves and repent, then our spirit aligns with the high frequency waves of life giving energy and our bodies begin to get well again.

32 But when we are judged, we are chastened of the Lord, that we should not be condemned with the world.

1 Cor 11:28-32 (KJV)

Sicknesses are meant to cause you to cry out to God for help. This is one reason I am against hospitals for Christians. They are suppose to seek God when they get sick, not a doctor. Your warning siren is your body. If it is sick it means that you most likely are sinning. God is doing us a favor by letting us know we are out of line with Him. Sickness is meant to humble us. He is trying to warn you that you are headed for hell. If you do not heed the Father you will be 'condemned' with the world. What has Churchianity done with this beautiful message and warning system of God? They pray for the surgeons hands and thank God for their illness so they can glorify him with their suffering. It is intentional hateful behavior. If God is glorified by your illness then lets make you really sick so He can have all the glory possible. Hypocrite! Your own heart condemns you. Sickness is a sign that the spirit is out of alignment with the source of Life it needs to survive. It means that it is time to examine the heart and start repenting.

I love a true story that one of my daughters told me. A young man found out he had cancer and was about to die. So he visited everyone he ever knew and sincerely apologized to them for everything his heart told him he had done wrong. Then, the young man returned to his doctor. The astonished doctor could not find the cancer. How would your life change if you truly faced your faults and repented? How many people put off the good that they should do, believing that they will have time tomorrow. What if that time never comes? If today were your very last day on earth, how would you spend it? If you knew that tomorrow you were going to face God and give an account for your life, what would you do right now? We are too caught up in this world and our lives may well be the price for doing such.

Who encourages us to forget Reality? Who draws us into their daydreams and fantasies that never come to pass nor could ever come to pass. Visions of fame, fortune, power, and glory. Demons reinforce the wrong in people. Their spirits are energy behind the evil we see. We are kind of like the switch and the light bulb and they are the electricity. We can't see them but they tend to light up the evil in us.

There are a lot of people who teach you how to get in touch with your 'dark' side. There are also groups that meet and 'let it all hang out' literally.... they do....nudity and all as they freely enjoy their demons. The stories of complete possession after behaving like this are astounding and plentiful. All who do such things will greatly regret it one day. For all sin comes with a price and directly accessing demons in such a free full manner just opens the doors to more demons and they will enter, them and their wicked friends, and they will 'love' you. That's how a person can easily go from oppression to possession.

True long lasting freedom only comes from knowing the truth and moving on His Spirit in you. All other attempts will be band aid patches at best. I will do exorcisms on occasion. They are sort of like the spiritual ambulance. I normally only do them if someone is about to die and they need more time....then I will cast out the unclean spirit so they have more time to repent.

Hopefully, by the time this book is out, I will be nearing the completion of some of my prayer cabins and be ready to hold conferences. Everyone should learn how to do proper exorcisms and know how to call up and command the demonic spirit safely and effectively.

I find that exorcisms can have a nasty side affect depending on how volatile the demonic spirit is. I've had some people stop breathing or go berserk, others sense nothing while the spirit watches me through their hosts eyes. You never know what will happen during an exorcism and for this reason the process will be taught at conferences.

Unclean spirits are at the helm of nearly all illnesses but they live and move within and according to our faults. If we cast them out we will heal the sick. However, you have to remove the fault to stay well. The Truth must be heard in the soul and heart for this to occur. No one can do it for you. It is something that you must seek with fear and trembling. It is that important. This is why we are to preach the gospel, the good news/the truth, to every person everywhere. Lies loved and known by man are killing him. We must tell people that they have to repent to enter heaven.

Sickness comes to those who move outside of Him. He is life. If you take a plant and pull it out of the sun into deep shade and darkness what happens to it? It begins to wither away and die. You are just like that. If you move from things like greed, lust, fear, selfishness, self pity, worry, doubt, anger, resentment, bigotry, pride, hate, perversion, etc. you will get sick. If you don't repent, move back into the sunshine, you will die.

I've had people point at wicked people and say, "but how come that person is alive. Look how bad they are yet they are 'very' healthy!" Sin has stages like cancer. At first you don't know it is there....but come back later and it will be fully evident. Not all sickness comes from sin. Jesus said so Himself. Some sins lead to accidents.

1 And as *Jesus* passed by, he saw a man which was blind from *his* birth.

2 And his disciples asked him, saying, Master, who did sin, this man, or his parents, that he was born blind?

3 Jesus answered, Neither hath this man sinned, nor his parents: but that the works of God should be made manifest in him.

John 9:2-3 (KJV)

It isn't helpful to get man's input on what is wrong with you. One must get the Truth from God and then when you move upon that truth from the right place in your heart, what can stop you from becoming well?

If you wish to grow healthier every day, the best way is to combat the demonic spirits in your life. This is done by simply seeking to close all the doorways. Stop drawing up hell in you and taking counsel with the demons to formulate the next piece of gossip, next ploy for attention, or greedy ambition. If you have to, stay away from people who draw you into sin. Mark the wicked man who loves to encourage you to mock others with him, belittling everyone and everything. Have you ever noticed what a kick demons get out of tormenting you through other people?

Start wising up to their schemes. Demon's love to play good cop bad cop with and in your mind. Most people never even see it. People assume they are having a conversation with God in them or with themselves and one or more devils are the inner voices they hear.

When someone hurts your feelings this is the first sign that your flesh is fully functional. Hurt feelings are like a red flare. Self is fully alive and doing well when you feel really 'sorry' for yourself. It is probably one of the most deceitful character traits that people have because it feels a lot like real humility, but isn't.

Tell me, if God is providing for all your needs according to His riches in glory why should I feel sorrow for your 'self'? Why should you feel sorry for yourself either? Don't you believe that God is keeping His word to you? Do you see the blasphemy here? Are you not complaining about Him when you feel sorry for you? What are you saying of His providing hand? All your needs encapsulates the physical and the spiritual. If you weren't using other people your feelings wouldn't get hurt. So who is the wicked one in that scenario?

Yes, the truth is hard to hear but the reward is huge! You don't have to feel sorry for yourself 'ever' again. You don't need anyone....honest! God is all that you need....forever. He will provide regardless of everything around you. He led you beside still waters, past tense. All that you need is already in Him. Read Psalms 23 in a new light and your soul will be blessed.

Self pity causes cancer and every person who lives from self pity will come and help you feel sorry for yourself. They are 'helping' you die. Are these people your real friends? Who is promoting wrong thinking and emotions in your life? Don't look for people to agree with you when you know you are wrong. Two wrongs never make a right. However, if you move on the wisdom that I just shared with you, that you really don't need anyone but God, if God opens that understanding up to you, you will be free from so much anger and frustration it will blow your mind away! That revelation will continue to grow if you don't let go of it and healing will come to your body.

It is our faults that get in the way of our healings. Paul said so and I know so. Unrepentant sin takes what should be a life of 120 years and whittles it down to 80 at best. We just don't listen to God. If we would only heed God. If we would only listen to Him when He tells us to not speak evil of others. Just that one thing would break so many demons from mankind that the health care businesses would have to start closing their doors.

It isn't that we need so much to train every person to cast out demons, but that we need to teach people what the price is for sinning.

Imagine a chart on the wall and on that chart all the days that you could live. Then, every time you sinned I marked a day off. If you could see me do that daily, how hard would you begin seeking God to be free from your faults so you could cease from sin? You cannot stop sinning on your own. Remember, only the Truth sets you free. You aren't the Truth. You have to ask God, "why am I doing this? Help me to stop? Show me, Lord I pray, and give me the strength to obey You. I want to honor Your name, not a demons! Dear God help me...!"

There are illnesses that come that are not from sin. Most are, but some are not. Please do not take liberties in judging others as to their illnesses. God is not pleased by this nor does He take pleasure in the suffering of mankind. Some things just wear out. The human body does. Teeth do too and so do joints and things. Paul spoke of these kinds of illnesses and so did Jesus and both said that God was more than willing and able to heal. The real problem is that people have lost their understanding and in doing so they have lost their faith in God. They think God sent them good doctors. This was not nor is it God's will for man. It is second best (or less) and I would certainly pray for mercy if you decide to go with man's ability to heal you.

Man was only designed to function a certain way to live in peace and wellness. If he moves outside of that way, he begins to die. His spirit actually begins to die.

Four

Churchianity

Man discovering himself as God....

Hold onto your hats and your pride this chapter
is going to be a bumpy ride if you love religion and
church. I'm going to expose your religion and your
church for what they are and what they are doing to
you spiritually. Hopefully you can be saved.

Church can be the worst place for you to go to
get to know God. They will invariably destroy the
discovery process in you and laden you with
burdens and guilt and destroy God in you. I want
you to understand that I am against organized crime.
I am against a hierarchy. And I am against anything
that destroys God/HF in people. There's nothing
quite like a man on an ego trip with a bible in his
hand. Their victims are many and they are generally
not ashamed of their sin.

Why are all religions nearly identical in format
and protocol? Who taught them all? Was it Jesus
who was rarely in the synagogue? Who has created
programs, titles, famous people, and worship of
buildings?

Your church owns you. I'm going to show you

how they are able to do that. Your heart tells you that I am right. If you are an 'important' person in the church you resent me for telling you the truth. If you are enslaved you are happy to read this where no one can see your great relief and you are secretly excited at the prospect of becoming free as you know not how to do it.

You are being brainwashed. It all began with an initial shock. If you were raised in church you may not even remember the incident(s) that began your slavery. In order to brainwash you you must first receive a deep emotional shock. Then you must continue to be shocked to stay brainwashed. This is the reason for the yelling from the pulpit and hell fire and damnation preaching. Once you have been given the picture of fear and received their 'salvation' they proceed to guilt trip you into obedience. None of this is God. It is man trying to control man to get the outcome he desires from you. The only way you can get relief from their pressure is to give in and appease those who 'lord' it over you. This is done by your church attendance, financial support, and volunteering. These make you a 'good' Christian and the clergy laud your spiritual growth which is really slavery. Those who become brainwashed must continue to receive shocks to stay brainwashed which is why they cannot stop going to church. These moments make them feel alive as they experience their shock(failing) over and over again.

Like I said, the next step in controlling you after the initial shock is to guilt trip you. Once you have been brainwashed/saved then they proceed to indoctrinate you so you cannot escape. Preachers and evangelist don't want you to know this. They wouldn't be able to pad their pockets, be worshiped, or enjoy their authority and mini god like status if you were to see the truth of what they are doing to you. It is considered one of the most lucrative easy career choices out there.

After awhile, you will not be able to miss church without extreme guilt. You will obey the 'church' and guess what? You belong to it. It doesn't belong to you, you belong to it. You will give it your money, your time, and your life. Your church has become your God. You serve it in Jesus name. Meanwhile, you die inside one sermon at a time as they horse whip you with God's precious words, spitting on you and demeaning you from the pulpit. Your mind forsakes you, falling asleep from the hypnotic influences. For heaven's sake, follow your mind and leave!

Your heart belongs to God, not the church. You are supposed to give it to the Truth, to Jesus. And while you play the church game all the while somewhere in the recesses of your heart and mind is this little nagging voice telling you something is horribly wrong. You can feel yourself being drained, robbed, and eaten alive. Emotionalism and fleshly games of importance, power, lust, and a promise of fame and glory is all you have left. You either play or get played. The proud play the game and usually get burned as there are only so many 'leadership' positions available. The meek get destroyed and are considered just 'laymen' or really food for the proud.

Do you honestly think that Jesus would go to churches as they are today? Do you really believe that Paul would have been agreeable with all the neat programs, advertisements, flag waving, paganism, and 'classes' that you see today? Your own heart convicts you. God is much greater than your heart. You take your children there and kill them too. What chance do they have to know the Truth when you destroy their discovery process with your rote memorization and Pharisee ways? May you wake up before it is too late for you or your little ones.

You see, God is the 'opposite' of religion. If you honestly want to be spiritual you need to realize that it will cost you your 'religious' friendships and ways. They can't go where you are about to go. They can't live day by day in the Truth. They cannot fathom watching spirits walk around, talking to God, and actually hunting down and destroying with passionate hatred any fault or sin that would keep one from growing closer to the Father. They don't give 10 percent...all that they have is His. They gave it all away the day they gave Him their life. They don't look for ways to impress people and be idolaters, they serve only the Living God. They are the church whereas the religious just play church.

Why have you not seen it? Pride blocked your view. You wanted to be important and you wanted to be special and loved. Silly you, you are already important, special, and loved because you belong to the Father. You don't need anyone else to see it for it to be real. Whatever made you think you weren't?

Are you willing to leave Egypt? Are you willing to lay down your ego? Can you stop playing church and serve God? If not, why are you wasting your time? You might as well seek the world altogether if you aren't going to serve God in the first place. Your punishment would be less severe than spending hours and hours listening to the Bible read to you while you love and live in your flesh.

You were not designed to discover the Truth from an outward place but inwardly, in your heart. You feel your heart burn even as I speak because I speak the Truth. The deeply religious and arrogant will not make it past this page. Their minds are too dark to hear me. Systematized religion kills more people than it helps. If you feel controlled by your church it is a warning sign. If you can't miss a service without the glare or questioning from a professional guilt tripper then get out! Leave before it is too late. Find God in the right way in your own heart and you will never need to be taught by man.

Churches never graduate anyone. Have you noticed? They create cripples who cannot move on their own because they must be stimulated from the outside instead of from the Holy Spirit on the inside. Once you are His it is all so easy to see but when you are caught up in the game of church it can be so dark and blinding. You find yourself needing everyone's approval and begin to live to their eyes. This breaks the first commandment of God! You will be miserable as you may well have noticed.

I am not saying not to gather with people who love God. I'm saying that most churches don't even know Him. When you gather with a group, look for one without fancy titles or pride abounding. Maybe even a home church or just a group of Truth lovers talking over a hot beverage. Look for people who honestly have God's character who aren't aspiring to become famous, important, or glorified. People with real hearts and real lives that want the same thing you do....the Truth. And the most important thing is ….do they honestly confess their faults to one another in sincerity? If they don't, they aren't interested in overcoming them.

Your pastor isn't your God and he or she, if they are a real pastor, will lay their life down for the others. This means that they don't do anything for themselves. They don't try to build up an image, get people to give them money, or get recognition. Jesus washed the feet of others. Surely a man should be that humble seeing that Christ our King was such a person. No pastor or teacher should have a mini throne, his/her own theme music, or be angered if you don't call them by their 'title' and such nonsense. If the pastor behaves like this, get out! They are being led by unclean spirits and do you want an unclean spirit to lead or teach you?

The group that you fellowship with should bear resemblance to God's own character. God is kind, humble, generous, forgiving, patient, and genuine. If you can't find a group like this you are markedly better alone. You will become your friends. Do not, I repeat, do not seek to fulfill any emotional needs through people. You have a God, remember? He takes care of 'all' your needs. This is His job and why He wants to be your God. Don't insult Him and try and replace Him with a little carving of wood or a friend named Pastor Bob.

God did send some people to His children. But don't you think that these people might act like Him in the earth? Jesus wore one set of clothing, was homeless, kind of heart, healed people, cast demons out, and told people to repent of their sins. If a minister of His is here, don't you think they might act like Him in the earth seeing that they are representatives of heaven? They probably aren't going to be flying around in their private jets. People follow these kind of religious folks because secretly they want a private jet too. Lust really blinds the eyes!

A pastor or teacher that is demonically led can do a lot of damage to your soul. Don't trade your soul for your flesh.

I'm stunned by how many preachers act like the

devil and say they are of God. Sorry folks, you are what you are. If you are God's, don't you think you might take on His nature at some point? If He is your teacher you are either a really bad student or not one at all. Think about this next time someone tries to destroy you while spouting out scriptures, condemning, and moving from arrogance, pride, and hate. Who are they kidding?! That is devil behavior all the way! If it looks like a duck, quacks like a duck, and walks like a duck....it's a duck.

Five

Death and Hell

The dimension nearest our own

One of the false doctrines we've looked at is that many churches teach is that human spirits are not unclean spirits because unsaved humans are all in hell. Let's see what the bible really says about death and hell and we'll also look at the motive behind the teaching. Where does this teaching come from? Is it correct and if not, why?

I realize that we all see in part and know in part, but if the part that you see is from the Holy Spirit it will remain true regardless of the other parts shown to you. You will find that when the Holy Spirit adds to what you have already been shown by Him it will never disprove what has already been imparted. Just as a diamond will always be a diamond no matter what size it is, so the truth will always remain true to itself as it is God who cannot change.

We know that death came to humanity through mankind's sin. Remember, sin is wrong thinking acted on. That is all it is.

21 For since by man *came* death, by man *came*

also the resurrection of the dead.
1 Cor 15:21 (KJV)

Death, the realm of the dead, came to this world by man. It is still the same today.

22 For as in Adam all die, even so in Christ shall all be made alive.
1 Cor 15:22 (KJV)

This means that something you or I are doing from birth that causes something to happen to us that kills us. When you are in Adam/LF (wrong thoughts) your mind and heart moves upon thoughts and ways that are not of God/HF. This is what it means to live and move in sin. All who live and move in this frequency range will die. Life (Christ) also comes through your being when you move upon His thoughts and ways/HF. All who live and move from God's thoughts, emotions, and ways will live.

1 This *is* the book of the generations of Adam. In the day that God created man, in the likeness of God made he him;

2 Male and female created he them; and blessed them, <u>and called their name Adam</u>, in <u>the day when they were created.</u>
Gen 5:1-2 (KJV)

God created mankind and called *them* Adam.....not in a singular sense. Look again at these verses:

21 For since by man *came* death, by man *came* also the resurrection of the dead.

1 Cor 15:21 (KJV)

Death/Darkness comes to you by mankind and through mankind comes Christ/Light. This is one way of saying that spirit flows through your being/spirit and creates your future. You have two sources to draw from or to follow. Those who are earthly are of Adam and those who are spiritual are of Christ. Paul is talking about 'types' of frequencies or walking two succinct paths which end in two different locations. Remember, God is all and in all and that He is the all Spirit God. This means that 'all' that you see is spiritual. Carnality is when the frequency vibrations are low and corrupted. Adam moved from a low frequency thought and all who are in him will die. Life comes from obedience to God/HF. This happens through confession and true recognition of low frequency thoughts and ways and repentance (turning from those ways). This is accomplished in Christ by repenting from the way you were living and happens when you give your self to His thoughts and ways. Once you commit your heart to live from the Truth instead of that which was not true you have been saved from death. This is salvation. As long as you are in Christ/Truth your LF's/sins that you are not aware of are covered by His blood. He is the one who gave His blood in the place of yours and died so you don't have to and only HF blood can restore LF blood. The key is that you must live according to His Mind in you and obedient to His voice within you and as long as you do there is no condemnation or LF returning upon you.

This energy behind all who are in 'Adam' are moving from and motivated by wicked spirits, either their own or others. Death came by man's disobedience to God or the Truth and obedience to another spirit. It is still the same process to this day. Life came to us also by a man, Jesus, who obeyed God and bore the sins of the world. Therefore, it is easy to see that Life has come to us through obedience to the Truth.

Death is a spiritual place and all physical conditions are spiritual ones. Death is a vibrational frequency. Again, ghosts who are the dead emit a very low frequency. The further you get from Truth, the lower your frequency. Eternal hell is the lowest frequency and creation has not stooped to it yet. Attacking Christ upon His return will invoke this frequency.

You can live in death and still have a body. If it were not so, then God lied and he can not. Adam became the 'dead', entered death by lowering his vibrations the moment he disobeyed God which is why he had to leave the garden. He could no longer exist in a HF world. Dimensions shifted and lowered and he found himself outside the garden/HF.

Let's look at what God told Adam:

"But of the tree of the knowledge of good and evil, thou shalt not eat of it: for in the day that thou eatest thereof thou shalt surely die.
Gen 2:17 (KJV)

God told Adam that in the _day_ that he would take good and evil into himself and acknowledge them both in him, that would be the day that Adam would know the realm of death in himself. This is the realm where the 'dead' go, the realm where all who 'believe' and love lies dwell whether they have a body or not. Adam went there the day he disobeyed God and his body lived on for several hundred years but began to age as it was from that moment on that he emitted low frequencies. You can not co-mingle God with something else and still obtain purity. The Truth cannot be diluted and still remain the Truth. Satan and evil spirits try to change the Truth and use Him to do their own dirty work. It is impossible for God to lie. It is impossible for High frequencies to lower. Man separates himself from God and begins his life on earth in this separated state as he is born into LF.

God goes on to explain that He brought Adam/mankind from a place before Life was given to him, and explains that this would be the place were Adam would return.

17And unto Adam he said, Because thou hast hearkened unto the voice of thy wife, and hast eaten of the tree, of which I commanded thee, saying, Thou shalt not eat of it: cursed *is* the ground for thy sake; in sorrow shalt thou eat *of* it all the days of thy life;

18 Thorns also and thistles shall it bring forth to thee; and thou shalt eat the herb of the field;

19 In the sweat of thy face shalt thou eat bread, till thou return unto the ground; for out of it wast thou taken: for dust thou *art*, and unto dust shalt thou return.

Gen 3:17-19 (KJV)

Here is how all curses come into your life. Take a close look as I explain. First, you move upon a thought that is incorrect and in the low frequency range. We give in to the voice/temptation because we wanted something. It may be the approval of a loved one, recognition, money, fame, or such things. Our lusts pulled us away from what we knew was correct and good. In that moment that we partook of the low frequency (forbidden fruit) and we emitted it. From then on things are cursed. You will never have enough. All you do will be consumed. You will have to fight for everything and obtain nothing and you will return to the place you got your knowledge from. Here is proof that the dead work to create the dead. The moment you bow your knee to them, that is the moment you become 'your friends'. Whatever you look to to fulfill your needs owns you.

How does death come to humans even now? It is still sin unto death and a person living in sin/wrong thinking acted on is as dead then as they are now. Basically, a person who lives for lies is dead while they speak and must be 'born again' or reborn unto Truth to live. Life comes from knowing the Truth in you. For it is faith or moral conviction in the Truth that causes repentance unto salvation.

Adam was told that he came from 'dust' and was going to return there. This dust is the realm of death, the great void or low frequencies. This void is the place where the dead are at right now. Satan is in the dust with the dead.

The bible says that the serpent was created by God and placed in the garden of Eden. It does not specify that God put the devil in the tree. Eve did that when she lusted after the fruit. Evil has no power to corrupt anyone, even now, unless you desire it and yield to it. It cannot destroy you if you don't allow it to enter you through your lusts.

"Now the serpent was more subtil than any beast of the field which the LORD God had made. And he said unto the woman, Yea, hath God said, Ye shall not eat of every tree of the garden?"

Gen 3:1 (KJV)

So we see that the Satan was already present. God had made the light and the darkness, good and evil, and Satan the serpent. God had put the tree in the garden to create His son's and daughters giving

99

them a choice to obey or disobey. Satan was not a threat to God's children although very present in the garden and created by God. It was Eve's lust for the fruit that brought evil to life. Thus, temptation's power comes from your own lusts and your corruption begins within your own heart aided by hell's fury.

And the LORD God said unto the serpent, Because thou hast done this, thou *art* cursed above all cattle, and above every beast of the field; upon thy belly shalt thou go, and dust shalt thou eat all the days of thy life: 15 And I will put enmity between thee and the woman, and between thy seed and her seed; it shall bruise thy head, and thou shalt bruise his heel.

Gen 3:14-15 (KJV)

Here we see that Satan had legs because he use to be a seraphim. He was able to travel into the heavens, but because of what he had done God **_removed_** his 'legs'. Satan lost his ability to move between the realms and was now grounded on his belly with the mess he had made—in the dust. Satan's actions lowered him in frequency. Many people do not realize that Satan is simply destroying himself.

Now look at the word 'dust' again. There is a deeper meaning to the word 'dust'. This particular word is what Adam and all mankind was created from before he was alive with the breath of God. Remember that God 'breathed' into Adam to give him life. Man's spirit is from God's Spirit. He is Life itself and our spirit is in His image. His Energy was like our energy before we fell from his frequency. The word dust represents the realm of death and low frequencies that our earthly bodies came from. Adam was brought forth from that which was not, just like the earth. Dust is nothingness, death, void, and emptiness. Those who do not know Life in them know death in them and to dust they return. Look at the way the word 'dust' is used again here in Isaiah.

"And thou shalt be brought down, *and* shalt speak out of the ground, and thy speech shall be low out of the dust, and thy voice shall be, as of one that hath a familiar spirit, out of the ground, and thy speech shall whisper out of the dust.
Isaiah 29:4 (KJV)

God was not talking about a spirit that was made evil just for the purpose of being evil. He is talking about the dead and the realm of dust or death. Satan is with the dead in the realm of low frequencies. Now compare it to this verse:

And when they shall say unto you, Seek unto them that have familiar spirits, and unto wizards that peep, and that mutter: should not a people seek unto their God? for the living to the dead?
Isaiah 8:19 (KJV)

101

Dead people speak out of the ground, the place of 'dust'. This is a place where you have to 'peep' into because it is not noticeable to the naked eye. Their speech is low or quiet and also refers to the frequency they operate in.

God didn't say to not contact fallen angels or Nephilims. He wasn't worried about that. He said don't seek the dead. The voices from the dust that whisper out of the ground that are familiar to us are the lost in the realm of death.

When you try to know and obey both truth/HF and lies/LF in you, your soul will return to the void from whence it came. Adam had an uncorrupted body but the moment he sinned it became corrupt. It wasn't heading for the dust until he sinned. Jesus bore a body of dust and He took his with Him as His sinless nature was not corrupt. Remember the spiritual law that spirit effects and controls matter. This dust is the realm of death where the 'dead' are at and the dust or basic elemental frequencies were used to create your body. Fallen angels and Nephilims are not the voices that psychics and soothe-sayers channel. Human spirits inhabit human bodies. It is that simple. It is hard to hear but it is absolute Truth.

Now, lets compare the description of 'dust' to Luke 11:24 and you will understand it.

When the unclean spirit is gone out of a man, he walketh through dry places, seeking rest; and

102

**finding none, he saith, I will return unto my
house whence I came out.**

Luke 11:24 (KJV)

Unclean spirits wander in the land of 'dust' which is why they try to relive their lives inside of people. The land of dust is a dry place. The Greek word used here for the word dry means without water. Dust, death, dry places, are all words used to describe the dwelling place of the dead, the place where mankind...all those who are in Adam (low frequencies) will return to the dust/LF; a place without the Living Water.

Let's continue to look at where God said Adam/mankind would go and where the bible actually says that the dead are at. Most theologians falsely teach that eternal hell is where all nonbelievers go when they die and that if you don't give your life to Jesus before you die it is too late, you are now in hell's eternal fires. They actually teach this false doctrine which has absolutely NO scriptural foundation. Here is what the bible actually says about death and the dead.

The word 'hell' is used in the bible for Sheol, the pit, Hades, and the grave. Notice that one dimension, heaven, is above the other, hell; this is referring to placement of dimensions and frequencies. Eternal hell is the one where all those who live in the low frequency range will go one day with the serpent and the false prophet and it has not even been created yet. Yet preachers are preaching that you go to a place of no return if you aren't saved and they have been teaching this false doctrine for centuries. Eternal hell is created for those who miss the second judgment. Come on folks, God is mercy. Do you think he's going to give up on His creation so easy? He is Wisdom. If there is a way to save your hide.....He'll find it!

Rev. 20:12 And I saw the dead, small and great, stand before God; and the books were opened: and another book was opened, which is *the book of life*: and the dead were judged out of those things which were written in the books, according to their works.

All the dead who were not saved will come together for 'another' great day of judgment. This is the second judgment. Those who are saved, are not present during the opening of this second book. God is still working with the dead. Why are people so quick to throw each other away? It's horrible and what is worse is the way the church uses the aspect of it to brainwash people, shocking people into fearful salvation prayers and using them to build buildings and pay their wages. I wouldn't want to be those hypocrites come judgment day!

The second book and day of judgment have no bearing on those who did truly give their lives to Jesus now and those who die trying to follow all that they know is right. These are those who are emitting HF. This second book is just for those who missed it the first time. These people are judged according to their works which means they are still 'working'. Although they did not emit HF upon death God will look at their over all record.

So here are the dead (those who did not give their lives to God who did not live within the high frequency range) both small and great, standing before God and the second set of books are opened. Everyone deserves a second chance, right? All the records of what they ever did, both while alive on earth and while in the realm of death, are opened and they are judged according to their 'works'. This will bring many who once knew God, but fell, into heaven's gates. This is wondrous news and when the main harvest is brought in! The first group saved are just the first fruits. In an orchard the first fruits are a very small portion of the fruit that come ripe. The big harvest comes later. So it is in heaven. Most people will be saved at the second judgment. God is most gracious and loves us alot.

We see in scripture that there is more than one dimension pertaining to heaven. Is Hades the same way? Yes, as the more degenerate you are the further you are from HF and the more painful it is because your spirit is being pulled apart. I'm sure it feels like burning.

2 I knew a man in Christ above fourteen years ago, (whether in the body, I cannot tell; or whether out of the body, I cannot tell: God

knoweth;) such an one caught up to the third heaven. 2 Cor. 12:2 (KJV)

Paul didn't know if this person had an 'out of body' experience or not but he knew that this person went and saw the third dimension in HF.

Paradise is the third dimension. It use to be lower and in or near Sheol which also has places or levels of dimensions or chambers. These are frequency levels. One could easily establish realms and worlds by set frequencies and vibrations, after all, all of creation as you know it are just vibrations. Everything is a vibration and so is heaven and hell. Just as a radio can bring in many stations, dimensions easily exist within the same space at the same time. So what we perceive spatially as up and down I see in my mind's eye as faster and slower, wider and narrower band width. The faster the vibrations the higher the dimension. In order to move dimensions or creation all that God must do is think of it and His thoughts produce the vibrations that cause the effect. Hence it would be nothing to move paradise to a different wave length or set of frequencies/vibrations. I use these words loosely to only represent my childlike concept of dimensions.

Let's take a look at some of the aspects of the realm of death and why I know that paradise was moved. Part of the reason that Jesus died and went to the belly of the earth was to change this dimension, but lets start at the beginning.

1 In the beginning God created the heaven and the earth.

We see two dimensions being created that affect one another and move in accordance to each other. We see what we recognize as spiritual (faster) and physical (slower).

2 And the earth was without form, and void; and darkness *was* upon the face of the deep. And the Spirit of God moved upon the face of the waters.

The physical world is about to come into form from the low vibrations, the face of the deep. The earth had no form....which translated means 'empty'. 'The face of the deep' means 'before'. And the translation of darkness means 'death'. Right now the realm of death is all that there is, it is empty, and God's Spirit is about to move and recreate a new heaven and a new earth. It is as if the earth and heavens and all creation is yet in the imaginative state of God's mind. He's thinking about doing it. Replacing the words with the base Greek meanings to the words used in the bible verses 1 through 2 would read something like this:

In the very first place, the very first moment of our time and our existence, God and His angels chose to make that which is air or not solid (the spiritual) and that which was solid or in other words, the physical.

Remember, all matter is not solid but vibrates. (Under a powerful microscope one can see through any matter.) Matter is made up of particles. Were they deciding the frequencies that would be used and the vibrations? Were the angels and God conversing about how to bring into being the next world?

1 And that which was physical, at the very beginning of time, was a place without purpose and was empty and obscure, and the realm of death was in but above the abyss/sea and was empty.

One creation had ended and they were thinking up the next.

2 The Spirit of God moved upon the what he saw and what was before Him.

He saw what was good to do and did it.

The realm of death is empty, the earth is without form and is void of inhabitants......Sound familiar?

Our age has an ending foretold which is soon to be upon us and God will once again confer with His angels and start anew. Will you or I be there planning the next earth? I think it is very likely.

The earth is like a garden. How many times has God created sons and daughters upon it? When everyone whose names are not written in the book of life are sent to eternal hell, Hades will be empty once again. Darkness and void upon the abyss. The bible says that God will create a new heaven and a new earth.....round and round it goes.

3 And God said, Let there be light: and there was light. 4 And God saw the light, that *it was* good: and God divided the light from the darkness.

Gen 1:1-4 (KJV)

God creates the realm of darkness or death, the void. Then from this void he creates the earth we live on. These are two dimensions that still effect each other. There are holding places for the dead, just as there are differing levels of heaven. Look at where the dead come from:

13 And the sea gave up the dead which were in it; and death and hell delivered up the dead which were in them: and they were judged every man according to their works.

14 And death and hell were cast into the lake of fire. This is the second death.

15 And whosoever was not found written in the book of life was cast into the lake of fire.

Rev 20:12-15 (KJV)

There are three places mentioned here that hold the dead; the sea, death, and hell. The lake of fire, eternal hell, is created at the end of the age of the earth and notice that the 'sea' remains and is later on spoken of as 'no more sea' while death and hell are thrown into the eternal pit. That means that its inhabitants are thrown into the internal inferno. This is when real eternal hell, the place of no return, begins. God is destroying these realms, including the realm of the sea.

1 And I saw a new heaven and a new earth: for the first heaven and the first earth were passed away; and there was no more sea.

Judgment takes place of the dead here at this time.

2 And I John saw the holy city, new Jerusalem, coming down from God out of heaven, prepared as a bride adorned for her husband. 3 And I heard a great voice out of heaven saying, Behold, the tabernacle of God *is* with men, and he will dwell with them, and they shall be his people, and God himself shall be with them, *and be* their God. 4 And God shall wipe away all tears from their eyes; and there shall be no more death, neither sorrow, nor crying, neither shall there be any more pain: for the former things are passed away.

Rev 21:1-4 (KJV)

The 'former' ways are gone. Death and the grave are gone and so is our earth. The lower frequencies and vibrations, spiritual and physical laws are brought to an end. This is what the demons will fight and attempt to keep from happening. Once it is gone, so are they. Praise the Lord! No more unclean spirits! No more dying and death will be forgotten. All the tears, all the pain, all the suffering, and torment will all be done away with as the new heaven and the new earth come into being. Who knows how many times God has done this! It is absolutely comforting to know that He knows exactly what He is doing and has done it thousands of times perhaps. The next Satan will be the first being to sin against full knowledge of the Truth.

1 And I saw an angel come down from heaven, having the key of the bottomless pit and a great chain in his hand.

2 And he laid hold on the dragon, that old serpent, which is the Devil, and Satan, and bound him a thousand years,

3 And cast him into the bottomless pit, and shut him up, and set a seal upon him, that he should deceive the nations no more, till the thousand years should be fulfilled: and after that he must be loosed a little season.

Rev 20:1-4 (KJV)

This place is the belly of the earth where Jesus went. Paradise, the resting place of those before Jesus' resurrection was also here in a chamber. Samuel, for instance, was brought up from the grave and David knew his spirit would go down to paradise but look at what Jesus told the man dying on the cross beside him.

And Jesus said unto him, Verily I say unto thee, To day shalt thou be with me in paradise.
Luke 23:43 (KJV)

Jesus told him that that very day he would be in paradise with him, yet where was he going?

For as Jonas was three days and three nights in the whale's belly; so shall the Son of man be three days and three nights in the heart of the earth.
Matt 12:40 (KJV)

Paradise was in the belly of the earth or else Jesus lied to that man on the cross. When Jesus died dead saints climbed out of their graves because they were released as paradise was in the process of moving upward in vibrations. They were simply passing through heading upwards.

50 , when he had cried again with a loud voice, yielded up the ghost.

51 And, behold, the veil of the temple was rent in twain from the top to the bottom; and the earth did quake, and the rocks rent;

52 And the graves were opened; and many bodies of the saints which slept arose,

53 And came out of the graves after his resurrection, and went into the holy city, and appeared unto many.

Matt 27:50-54 (KJV)

They came up 'after' his resurrection. Jesus set them free....bodies and all! We see here that the saints were sleeping just like Samuel. They also ascended but went to the third heaven to await the return of Christ and I'm sure Samuel was amongst them! How awesome! What else did Jesus do while in the belly of the earth?

18 For Christ also hath once suffered for sins, the just for the unjust, that he might bring us to God, being put to death in the flesh, but quickened by the Spirit:

19 By which also he went and preached unto the spirits in prison;

20 Which sometime were disobedient, when once

113

**the longsuffering of God waited in the days of
Noah, while the ark was a preparing, wherein
few, that is, eight souls were saved by water.**
                                    1 Peter 3:18-20 (KJV)

God had this plan when he flooded the earth. He
needed to clean up the mess that the giants had
made and so he had to wipe out the genetic
mutations. Was the only genetically pure race left on
earth that respected Him Noah and his family?

 Did God give up on people? No, he showed
them the Truth. He sent a rescuer to them and
preached the Truth to them and saved them in hell.
God doesn't give up on us, even when we do. He
will work with people through the 1,000 years,
showing them the truth, talking to them. He loves
His creation. He loves you. Your problems are never
too big for Him and He has more patience then
you'll ever dream of. His ways are beyond your
comprehension and He wants to live and dwell with
you forever. This is His desire. All might and
strength are His. I think He is more then able to save
humanity.

It reminds me of the old saying, 'we can do this
the easy way or the hard way'. God can go either
way. He's more time then you can imagine as He
sits outside of time itself. Your life span on earth is
but a moment to Him. I think He is able to endure
our misgivings. Jesus died for the sins of the 'whole'
world and that includes all people; people on all

vibrational frequencies. He didn't die in vain.

Lets look again at what Paul said about paradise:

2 I knew a man in Christ above fourteen years ago, (whether in the body, I cannot tell; or whether out of the body, I cannot tell: God knoweth;) such an one caught up to the third heaven. 2 Cor 12:2 (KJV)

This person went up, not down. After Jesus left the earth we see it recorded that paradise is up, not down as it use to be and is no longer in the belly of the earth.

In Revelations the Spirit says:

7 He that hath an ear, let him hear what the Spirit saith unto the churches; To him that overcometh will I give to eat of the tree of life, which is in the midst of the paradise of God.

Rev 2:7 (KJV)

A person who overcomes this world moves upward not downward proving that after the resurrection Paradise was moved to a higher vibration. Before, people could not ascend. Therefore, God had created a quiet place of rest in Hades for them but they could view the dead and hear the suffering. Now we have Jesus to remove sin from us. We are now able to overcome death and ascend, if we live for Him and not ourselves.

What about the other end of the spectrum? What happens in the lowest frequency range. Is this the lowest hell; the pit? The beast and the plague of locusts spoken of in Revelations comes out of the bottomless pit. These are higher ranking demons, not unclean spirits. I believe that this is the place referred to as the center of the earth where Jesus went upon His death and is what most Christians mean when they say 'hell'. I also believe that this is the holding tank of many of the dead and very possibly that which is referred to as the sea. There will be no need for this sea anymore without any dead and so it is done away with.

20 When I shall bring thee down with them that descend into the pit, with the people of old time, and shall set thee in the low parts of the earth, in places desolate of old, with them that go down to the pit, that thou be not inhabited; and I shall set glory in the land of the living;

Ezek 26:20 (KJV)

Lets compare that with **Isa. 29:4**

"And thou shalt be brought down, *and* shalt speak out of the ground, and thy speech shall be low out of the dust, and thy voice shall be, as of one that hath a familiar spirit, out of the ground, and thy speech shall whisper out of the dust.

The low parts of the earth are desolate, dry, dust, parched, and hot. They speak in a low voice like a whisper, meaning that they are distant but yet can be heard when strained or tuned in to. A thought so quiet that you might think it your own.

A pit was used to hold prisoners. Many exorcists send spirits to the pit during an exorcism and the spirits will beg to not have to go there like they did to Jesus saying, "it is not our time." All unclean spirits have a time frame that they operate in concerning their ability to enter the living. According to exorcisms this appears to be 120 years according to God's promise in Gen. 6:3 which was never altered by God although God in His mercy could certainly send or allow unclean spirits to stay or be bound as He sees fit. The pit is the lowest created frequency at this time. I have noticed in Muslim exorcisms that the time line is also confessed by the unclean spirit.

In the bible an earthly pit was used to hold criminals. It was firm on all sides and it nearly separated you from the living. It was cold, dark, and lonely and one who was its prisoner lived in the worst conditions. Death, Hades, Sheol, the Pit, the Sea, are all descriptions of where the dead are at. Could are differing levels of frequencies? Is Satan stuck in an extremely low frequency? He most certainly is because he is more degenerate than most other spirits having moved upon wrong thoughts longer and the most degenerate ways and fell the furthest as he was the nearest to God. This would

117

also explain why the fallen angels are bound, they are stuck there too, unable to transcend and ascend. What crime was so low that it locked them into that low of a frequency? It was the murder of Jesus Christ. Satan lost his legs and ability to traverse dimensions in the garden of Eden, he lost even more ability upon the murder of Christ which was more sin and with that sin comes the price....lower frequencies.

What profit *is there* in my blood, when I go down to the pit? Shall the dust praise thee? shall it declare thy truth?
Psalms 30:9 (KJV)

Will the 'dust' praise thee? Living Water is not in the pit. Sheol is a dry place, a place with less of God's life giving energy. Your works follow you and you will be judged by them. In other words, your frequency or spirit vibrations are really low, but how low? This would bring a cold feeling to you as your vibrations and oscillations slowed down. It would then begin to feel like burning as you get further and further away from the correct vibration. Is eternal death the moment you nearly stop vibrating? This would bring extreme pain to your spirit. The further you move from His vibrations the more you will suffer. People are sending themselves to hell and their suffering is due to their own actions.

118

Unto thee will I cry, O LORD my rock; be not silent to me: lest, *if* thou be silent to me, I become like them that go down into the pit.

Psalms 28:1 (KJV)

If the Truth, the correct vibrations, becomes silent to your own spirit, guess what vibration level your spirit has? How can it not go down to the pit? You are like an emitter station. If you don't have God's vibrations to move upon, whose do you have left? All that will come from your being will be corrupt.

The dead aren't far away in a fire named hell like the church falsely teaches they are close to you in a cold place that is so cold it burns them. They are in a dimension that merges with our own on low frequency levels. The lower they are, the further they are from the earth. They begin on our level and descend.

Dust or dirt was always a sign of death in the old testament. People would put dust on their heads to show that they were near death while in grief.

"And when they lifted up their eyes afar off, and knew him not, they lifted up their voice, and wept; and they rent every one his mantle, and sprinkled dust upon their heads toward heaven."

Job 2:12 (KJV)

It was man's way of telling God that he understood that he was nothing and it was an act of humility. God, who cannot lie, said that man would return to 'dust'.

19 God *is* not a man, that he should lie; neither the son of man, that he should repent: hath he said, and shall he not do *it*? or hath he spoken, and shall he not make it good?

Num 23:18-19 (KJV)

It is 'impossible' for God to lie. He cannot do it. He is the Truth. David said of the coming of the Messiah:

15 My strength is dried up like a potsherd; and my tongue cleaveth to my jaws; and thou hast brought me into the dust of death. 16 For dogs have compassed me: the assembly of the wicked have inclosed me: they pierced my hands and my feet.

Psalms 22:15-16 (KJV)

Jesus was about to be brought into hell for three days and three nights. As he began to die he says of the one's responsible that they were dogs and the assembly of the wicked. These were the spirits behind the scene. Jesus is saying through David, "they brought me into the dust of death". Hades/Sheol is the dust of death. In verse 29 it speaks of the dogs or demons that were behind the murder of the son of God and says.....

17 I may tell all my bones: they look *and* stare upon me.

18 They part my garments among them, and cast lots upon my vesture.

19 But be not thou far from me, O LORD: O my strength, haste thee to help me.

20 Deliver my soul from the sword; my darling from the power of the dog.

This was the prayer of Jesus spoken of through the mouth of David; a foretelling of future events that would one day take place. The 'power' or energy of the dog/devil is clearly seen as the ones who killed Jesus. Jesus then goes on to pray:

21 Save me from the lion's mouth: for thou hast heard me from the horns of the unicorns.

22 I will declare thy name unto my brethren: in the midst of the congregation will I praise thee.

23 Ye that fear the LORD, praise him; all ye the

seed of Jacob, glorify him; and fear him, all ye the seed of Israel.

24 For he hath not despised nor abhorred the affliction of the afflicted; neither hath he hid his face from him; but when he cried unto him, he heard.

God hears and responds positively to everything that comes from a right place in your heart. All that is right and good is Him in you. Every time you move from a correct thought or emotion, God hears you in a way that brings His answer to your prayers.

He hears the wicked, but the way he hears them is to answer them with his law of judgment. Devils bring the answers to all who move from evil thoughts and ways. This is God's judgment for the wicked of heart.

25 My praise *shall be* of thee in the great congregation: I will pay my vows before them that fear him.

26 The meek shall eat and be satisfied: they shall praise the LORD that seek him: your heart shall live for ever.

27 All the ends of the world shall remember and turn unto the LORD: and all the kindreds of the nations shall worship before thee.

28 For the kingdom *is* the LORD'S: and he *is* the governor among the nations.

Jesus is Lord because He took on the stucture of a human being and overcame LF's, all who are in Him will live forever. All that praise Him praise God as He is at one with God and in essence is God. Look at what is written next.

29 All *they that be* fat upon earth shall eat and worship: all they that go down to the dust shall bow before him: and none can keep alive his own soul.

Those who grow fat upon the earth are those who love God's ways. These are the only ones that will know God's blessings as they partake of His nature...His blood and flesh. Only those who examine themselves and turn from wrong thinking will be able to enter heaven and grow fat or be blessed. This happens now. You are right now either in heaven and hell. Your physical death is only the bus ride to your currant destination. Please realize that when your body dies your spirit simply goes to be with the one it loves and listens too. Who are you loving and listening too? Is it the truth; all that you know is right and good? If not, then there is only one other destination for the bus to stop. This bus stops at a place you don't want to go. These are they who move upon and love low frequency thoughts, ways, and emotions. These people love to feel sorry for themselves, hate others, relish in gossiping and slander. They just couldn't give up their ego's and love of self. These go into 'the dust' because no one can keep their own soul alive and only HF has life in it.

What is death? Death is the place where you cease or nearly cease to vibrate. All who begin to move on low frequencies are dying and in death because you are beginning your journey away from life/correct vibrations.

25 My soul cleaveth unto the dust: quicken thou me according to thy word.

Psalms 119:25 (KJV)

We can only be restored through knowing Truth in us, by having Him as the Lord of our lives, and living unto Him.

I think it is also important to point out that Satan doesn't consider the dead non useful. They aren't down there sleeping or lying quietly in their graves.

9 Hell from beneath is moved for thee to meet *thee* at thy coming: it stirreth up the dead for thee, *even* all the chief ones of the earth; it hath raised up from their thrones all the kings of the nations   Isaiah 14:9 (KJV)

I want you to see that the dead are still working,

124

doing, and for the majority, not in a nice way. Notice that Hell isn't stirring up the Nephilims or the fallen angels. How does it feel to know that Hitler may have risen in rank and could be a large part of what happens to people in the last days? There are many like him in hell. They are all planning to destroy God and all those who love Him. The battle of Armageddon is soon to come. Many of the dead will be there.

Tartarus, the pit, is the lowest part of the realm of death or the furthest away from our dimension.

12 How art thou fallen from heaven, O Lucifer, son of the morning! *how* **art thou cut down to the ground, which didst weaken the nations!**

Through the assault upon Jesus Satan moved lower. Afterward he saw his mistake, but it was too late. Lust drew him aside to kill Jesus; he saw his chance to become God. First, he tried to give Jesus the dominions and all that he ruled in the low frequency he was in, but Jesus, who was the Truth, of course did not accept the offer knowing that it didn't belong to Satan but only to God. Jesus quoted the truth to Satan (this is how all wrong thinking will be overcome in you.) Jesus' morals weren't corrupt. Later, Jesus was murdered and taken to hell by Satan's minions as they 'assumed' that Jesus had sinned believing that this was why they were allowed to finally access him and kill him. This is what fooled the devils. They were not permitted to touch Jesus before and now that they had, they just figured that Jesus had finally sinned. Here is what Jesus said:

17 Therefore doth my Father love me, because I lay down my life, that I might take it again.

18 No man taketh it from me, but I lay it down of myself. I have power to lay it down, and I have power to take it again. This commandment have I received of my Father.

John 10:16-18 (KJV)

No man could take Jesus' life away from him. The devils had been trying to kill him repeatedly and failed time after time in their ambitions. When they finally had their way with him, mocking, striking, and tormenting his flesh....they killed him believing it was because of their own wisdom and power that they had done it. They could not see what Love would do as they have no Love in them. They are corrupt as they only have only low frequency thoughts to move from and cannot know Wisdom in them. They could not perceive that Jesus would lay down His life for others. Devils cannot think HF thoughts. All God's plans are safe and secure for devils/LF minds cannot perceive the things of God.

7 But we speak the wisdom of God in a mystery, *even* the hidden *wisdom*, which God ordained before the world unto our glory:

8 Which none of the princes of this world knew: for had they known *it*, they would not have crucified the Lord of glory.

1 Cor 2:7-8 (KJV)

Had Satan known what was about to happen to his kingdom, his frequencies, he would have left Jesus alone. That is a strong statement! Jesus was leading people into the truth by the droves while walking around on planet earth, casting out unclean spirits, and healing multitudes!

When Jesus entered the lower frequency range it could not hold Him! He could enter because he had a human body which was corrupt but LF couldn't hold him because he was without sin/LF. He went to hell on his own accord, but being without sin/without a low frequency in him hell could not hold him. He spoke the truth to those in hell and many believed and came up from low frequencies to the higher ones! In His Light they saw Light! Jesus could have left the earth at any given time like Enoch. His life/correct frequencies were in him. Instead, he chose to die for you and I, in our place upon a cross. He bore the sins of many to redeem mankind. The reason? Love always does what is best for others. **He is pure love.**

What were the keys that he stole? We know that Jesus destroyed the veil or that which stood between us and God. We know that he died for our low frequencies and is now the one who speaks in our behalf before the throne of God but he did another important thing. He took away Satan's ability to lock up humanity. He overcame low frequencies! Then he gave us authority to cast out any spirit that moves upon them in others. Satan, sinned again, broke the law of God and moved into a lower frequency than he was already in! This made earth farther from his greedy grasp.

Satan could not see this plan because it comes from a place of Love. Satan and demons move from and upon low frequency thoughts. They are motivated by hate, lust, greed, strife, anger, vengeance, arrogance, pride, and love of self. They did not see Jesus' willingness to give His life for others, enduring the cross, the shame, and the torture all to help mankind in his struggle against low frequencies. This is one reason they were so brutal. They thought that Jesus would save Himself as He had always done if He was indeed sinless. Instead, Jesus chose to die. This was something demonic minds could not perceive. The same situation exists today in mankind. Those who are Christs are not understood by the world. Worldly minds cannot perceive how a person could not live for things and for themselves. How can you be happy being and having nothing? We are a mystery to the minds that dwell in the dark.

Here we see Satan's heart:

13 For thou hast said in thine heart, I will ascend into heaven, I will exalt my throne above the stars of God: I will sit also upon the mount of the congregation, in the sides of the north:

This is amazing because God actually lets us know that Satan had a dimension he was trying to overcome before the crucifixion—the sides of the North. He was leading 1/3 of heaven's fallen host trying to ascend even higher. He saw the fallen angels as his own army and believed he was becoming something amazing. How many people do you know that are busy becoming amazing?

14 I will ascend (in frequencies) **above the heights of the clouds; I will be like the most High.**

He was climbing the corporate ladder! Now I know the spirit behind the business world we see today. God had another result for Satan's lofty selfish ambitions.

15 Yet thou shalt be brought down to hell, to the sides of the pit.

Again, more wisdom imparted. The pit, the

center of the earth has 'sides' or chambers that restrict it. These are the principalities and powers that God has made, the rules by which creation works.

16 They that see thee shall narrowly look upon thee, *and* **consider thee,** *saying, Is* **this the man that made the earth to tremble, that did shake kingdoms;**

The word 'man' in Hebrew translated actually means 'person'. Is this the person that made the earth tremble? That will be the question asked! When they take a look at Satan they will realize he is a big nothing! If Satan had looked at himself correctly he would have seen it himself and never fallen. We are all nothing. God is everything. We cannot become something of ourselves because 'it doesn't exit'. Pride is a strong belief in something that simply doesn't exist. How many lives will be wasted on the lie that there is an existence outside of all.

17 *That* **made the world as a wilderness, and destroyed the cities thereof;** *that* **opened not the house of his prisoners?**

They will be astonished at the disgusting sight of Satan who tried to keep and use all the dead to do his dirty work. This worm who spent what time he had left destroying everything he could will be seen for what he is. His angry heart trying to become something that doesn't exist will one day be exposed. Meanwhile, his beauty that he once fell in love with begins to dwindle with each shift in frequency as the lower your frequency, the more grotesque the form as your spirit is stretched by the shift in frequencies. A fallen angel I saw had nearly lost all resemblance to anything remotely beautiful. They have been seen by many and are what people think of as aliens. They are the greys. That story will be on my website.

18 All the kings of the nations, *even* all of them, lie in glory, every one in his own house.

19 But thou art cast out of thy grave like an abominable branch, *and as* the raiment of those that are slain, thrust through with a sword, that go down to the stones of the pit; as a carcase trodden under feet.

They are tossed out of the grave and go to the pit. This also proves two separate places in what we commonly term 'hell'.

20 Thou shalt not be joined with them in burial, because thou hast destroyed thy land, *and* slain thy people: the seed of evildoers shall never be renowned.

Is. 14:9-20 (KJV)

After the second judgment, God will not bring

the wicked who love lies and practice lies lovingly back to life. They will join Satan in eternal hell after the thousand years are finished FOREVER. Today people are reknown. They are the unclean spirits who relive their lives through other people. In the future, this will come to an end.

Remember, God cannot lie. He has allowed mankind to stay in this dimension regardless of whether they have a body or not because the earth itself groans for redemption from being placed into the realm of death. Death reigns on earth and is only overcome in Christ. Once death and hell are thrown into eternal hell God is going to make a new heaven and a new earth and start all over. Again, will we be the ones to help? Is that why He is making us kings (those who have truth and rule over lies) and priests(those who help others see the truth)? What wonders our Father has for us to discover......I can't wait...!

Six

The Apocrypha
And other books of significance............

Among other important writings, I would like to
bring to light information concerning the dead
included in the sacred writings of the Apocrypha
which, by the way, was in the bible until 1611 and
contains many spiritual insights. Some people
confuse the Apocrypha with the Lost Books of the
Bible; these are entirely different and separate
writings and in my opinion, they bear more
credibility than many of the Lost Books. The
disciples quoted the Apocrypha and considered it
worthy enough to quote and so do I. It contains
much wisdom and I highly recommend it to be read
by every person in search of Truth.

In the Apocrypha, 2 Esdras, it clearly states that
the dead are wandering around the earth, not
floating in a pool of slime in the belly of the earth as
commonly depicted in movies. Jesus and the
disciples knew full well who unclean spirits/ghosts
were as the Apocrypha was a part of the bible of
their day and the Jews call the unclean spirits the
'dybukk' and still do to this day. Here is what the

Apocrypha has to say concerning the dead.

78 But now to speak of death: when the Most High has pronounced final sentence for a person to die, the spirit leaves the body to return to the One who first gave it, that it may render adoration to the glory of the Most High.

79 As for those who have scornfully rejected the ways of the Most High, who have spurned his law, and who hate the godfearing, their spirits enter no settled abode, but from then on must wander in torment, endless grief, and sorrow. And this for seven reasons.

2 Esdras 7:78-79(REB)

There is a reason why God inflicts punishment in a seven fold fashion. I will explain in detail at the end of this book. For now, lets just look at the fact of who unclean spirits are, where they are at, and the frequencies they move on.

Notice that God moves on the Highest Frequency (Most High). When He determines it is time for you to be removed from the vibrations/oscillations of the earth, He will move you on. This will either be an upward move for you or a downward move depending upon what frequency you have become while inhabiting your body and what is best for others and yourself. In theology this is known abstractly as heaven and hell. You determine your own fate by what you emit. No flesh will be glorified in His presence because it is all operating on a corrupt frequency. How can corruption honor God? Therefore it will be removed as it should and all of God's children will receive bodies that are incorrupt.

There is no 'settled' abode for unclean spirits. Their fate is to wander which is why they seek to live in others as they have no home anymore. They are wanderers, living in torment, and endless grief and sorrow because they didn't choose God's ways, His frequencies, while they had a body. They chose lies over the truth in them and they hated those who would tell them otherwise, those who dared to live according to the truth. Their lives were wasted on that which was not true and founded upon the false belief that there is existence outside of God. They followed the lies to the grave and when their bodies died their spirits remain in the frequency range they were emitting.

Ghosts are unclean spirits which are the souls of the dead. When you look at the word ghost you can see it being used interchangeably for spirit throughout the bible—Holy Spirit and Holy Ghost. Clean ghosts/spirits go to be with Lord and unclean ghosts/spirits remain in the earth on varying levels of corrupt frequency. The bible means exactly what it says when it says that unclean spirits enter people and must be cast out.

What happens to the saved? When a person dies, if they are saved, they go to be with the Truth/Lord because they are emitting high frequencies. Upon death they enter the realm of higher frequencies.

8 We are confident, *I say*, and willing rather to be absent from the body, and to be present with the Lord.

2 Cor 5:8 (KJV)

Hades or Sheol, the realm of death, is the destination of the dead. This realm is near or just below the realm earth, crossing over it in dimensions. This is why we are able to easily contact the dead. They are able to observe us more easily than we can observe them. We have bodies (settled abodes) but they do not which is why they are not tied down and are airborne. The Pit is the center or deepest lowest frequency away from earth. As a spirit lowers in frequency it becomes trapped within those frequencies and cannot ascend but can only descend. As it deteriorates spiritually it becomes confined to its frequency. It cannot move upwards to heaven as it cannot vibrate high enough. It appears that after 120 years their frequency is automatically lowered by God.

Light/HF actually hurts them and is painful to them. Their day of reckoning has already been set, the second judgment, and they are being reserved for that day. God is just and fair. Again, an unclean spirit is a spirit that has not been 'cleansed' by God or Truth. It does not vibrate on an acceptable level. It is a spirit that is being fathered by Satan/low frequencies, not God's Mind/high frequencies, and is therefore full of corruption and cannot occupy heavenly places. When psychics say that some spirits have ascended to the light, they are partially correct. The ascending happened before the death of their body and not afterwords. Again, psychics will say, "they went on to the light" and yes, they did, in that God is that Light and all who dwell in the Light cannot be reached by anyone in this dimension. There is a great gulf between those in the 3rd heaven and those in the realm of death.

24 And he cried and said, Father Abraham, have mercy on me, and send Lazarus, that he may dip the tip of his finger in water, and cool my tongue; for I am tormented in this flame.

25 But Abraham said, Son, remember that thou in thy lifetime receivedst thy good things, and likewise Lazarus evil things: but now he is comforted, and thou art tormented.

26 And beside all this, between us and you there is a great gulf fixed: so that they which would pass from hence to you cannot; neither can they pass to us, that *would come* from thence.

Luke 16:24-26 (KJV)

The word 'gulf' in Greek is the word 'chasma' meaning chasm or vacancy. This is the description of what once lie between the place where paradise was and the realm of death. God separated the two with an impassible barrier then, just think of how far away it is now that paradise has been moved. I believe that the two cannot view one another anymore.

I was always under the impression that there was a great difference between truth and lies and the Holy Spirit revealed to me while writing this that there is 'nothing' between a truth and a lie for all thoughts and emotions either are or are not of Him. That place that people try so hard to create, their own world, mixing a little bit of truth with a lie to get what their corrupt self wants...... this place doesn't exist. Evil is evil and good is good. They cannot be intertwined or co-mingled and a little sin leavens the whole lump/being.

God and creation has seven overall dimensions (frequencies or set of vibrations) upwards and downwards, each representing God's own Spirit and how we are made in His image. This is why seven is the sum of perfection. God's own spirit has seven aspects which I will describe at the end of this book.

There also appears to be a one week period in which a human spirit can be brought back to life into their bodies. God considers a person at the time of death to be 'sleeping' or dormant to their physical bodies/vibrations on earth. I'm going to show this to you from two points for you to consider.

11 He that toucheth the dead body of any man shall be unclean seven days. Num. 19:11 (KJV)

We see the time line here of when a spirit could still linger in a body to re-enter it to live again. After the seven days were up, the body can no longer 'house' the spirit(s) in it.

I asked him: 'When souls are separated from their bodies, will they be given the opportunity to see what you have described to me?

101 "They will be allowed seven days," he replied: 'for seven days they will be permitted to see the things I have told you, and after that they will join the other souls in their abodes.'

2 Esdras 7:100-101

There isn't just one abode or one frequency....but many sets of low frequencies. Spirits often stay near their body, like at graveyards, after entering the realm of death in their abode/frequency. I believe that the only good they can do anymore is to stay away from people and wait for their judgment in remorse. They are diseased. No matter how they enter a living person they kill them as they are in the low frequency range, bringing corruption with them where ever they go.

In some parts of Africa, a dead body is often left alone for many hours before it is prepared for burial. Black majick has the common practice of transferring demons into people via a witch doctor. It is commonly known that if you deal with a dead body too soon one will receive an electric shock from the unclean spirits and other spirits as they exit the corpse. To reduce the risk of demonic entry the dead are not touched for a certain period of time.

Also, demons can stay with organ donations. During and after transplants of a live tissue or organs an unclean spirit is able to move into the next person and suddenly you have grandmas who take up smoking and car racing after receiving a heart transplant from a young man. The grandma became the young man. It is easy to see where the character changes came from as this spirit enjoyed his new home. It is disturbing, to say the least, that people do not even realize what is going on.

Just as we do not know the names of the the heavens except the third one 'Paradise', the bible only mentions several names of the places of Darkness. Death, Hades, the Sea, Sheol, and the Pit are a few of the places in Darkness that the bible says that the dead go to and dwell at.

After seven days the human spirit enters the next

dimension to stay there till the second judgment, that is, if they are not moving at high frequencies. If they have drawn closer to Truth/God and seen their sin and repented, putting God first place in their life, then they ascend upwards. If they have drawn away from the Light in this world then they go to be with their kind and go downward into the dark that they loved while in their body and commence to wander the earth in spirit form in dusty dry places of torment.

Death is the final adventure of your physical life and vibrational experience that you had on earth. Your destination is very predictable however, if you know how death works. You simply go to be with the one you love and serve. You can only serve right or wrong, truth or lies. Although you can emit high or low frequencies intermittently you cannot love and follow Jesus/similitude of God and love and follow lies no more than one can turn to the left and the right at the same time. Serving yourself is serving that which is wrong and believing in oneself is a mistake that many souls make which will cost them everything. There really is only one God and it isn't you or I. We aren't that Light but can only be a vessel for the Light and bear witness of Him.

It is here in Job that you will see a direct comparison to human spirits as unclean.

13 But the hypocrites in heart heap up wrath: they cry not when he bindeth them. 14 They die

in youth, and their life *is* among the unclean.
Job 36:13-14 (KJV)

Did you see that? Hypocrites die and their life is among the unclean. They are among the 'unclean' spirits. Ghosts are unclean spirits. Have you ever noticed how people that channel them become very pale and sick after a while? Unclean spirits make you sick because they are 'low frequency'. Jesus healed people by casting them out. This is what every believer has the ability to do in Christ. It is imperative for every person to understand the world that they are in and the worlds that they are headed to. Ghosts often try to communicate using many means outside of human bodies but they offset our own frequencies just enough that manifesting in a form we can see is challenging but certainly not impossible as we have noticed. They have no bodies of their own anymore and can only enter this dimension in a feeling way through someone elses spirit vibrations. Also, should they reveal themselves and their intentions, who would let them stay? Would people knowingly invite death into them? This is why stealth is their biggest weapon and one of the reasons I am writing this book. I hope it saves your life.

Part of me is reluctant to share how easy it is for us to communicate with the dead because many people would rather perish with their dead loved ones then give their lives to God and the thought of never seeing certain family members again is too much for many to bear. They think that a dead loved one is the same person that they knew on this side of life and it is hard for them to understand that visitation and cohabitation is forbidden by God.

24 Verily, verily, I say unto you, Except a corn of wheat fall into the ground and die, it abideth alone: but if it die, it bringeth forth much fruit.

You have to die to this world's frequencies. Every thought, way, and action that comes from corrupt emotion and thinking must cease to exist in you for you to truly become alive.

25 He that loveth his life shall lose it; and he that hateth his life in this world shall keep it unto life eternal.

If you really cared for your own well being you would abandon the ways, thoughts, and emotions that are not of God. You must come to a place where you hate the ways of this world, knowing that they indeed bring death to your soul and the souls of others.

26 If any man serve me, let him follow me; and where I am, there shall also my servant be: if any man serve me, him will *my* Father honour.
                              John 12:23-26 (KJV)

You can only be a servant of Jesus if you *follow* Jesus. That means that you will be acting like Him and thinking His thoughts, speaking His words, and be a continuation of His presence in the earth. It has nothing to do with the type of clothes you wear, the church building you enter, the title you give yourself, or the amount of head knowledge you manage to acquire. These actions belong to the Pharisees. Salvation is a matter of the heart. Who does your heart serve. Whoever you serve, you follow. Who are you following? Do you serve the Truth or do you serve yourself? Are you proud, boastful, envious, cruel, angry, spiteful, hateful, or greedy? If you live from these emotions, then you serve the devil.

Wherefore, my beloved, as ye have always obeyed, not as in my presence only, but now much more in my absence, work out your own salvation with fear and trembling.
Phil 2:12 (KJV)

Unclean spirits are people who missed it. They are the ones who believed in themselves, spent their lives pleasing their flesh (corrupt frequencies), and loved the thoughts and ways that were incorrect. Contacting the dead in an inquisitive or loving manner will destroy you. Case after case of Ouija board user horror stories have not stopped people from purchasing it or the company from producing

144

the game. Arrogance says, "I am different...it won't happen to me. I control myself." It lies. Unclean spirits live strongly and easily in people who are proud. The proud are just more fully convinced of the lie that a power can exist outside of God who is all. This gives the demon more room to make you think you are the voices in your head. Therefore they can easily steal your life away and make and mold you into their own likeness and all the while you think you are becoming something....and yes, you are, just not the something that you foolishly believe! You are becoming fully dead.

People love to discover 'themselves'. They congregate with the dead knowingly and unknowingly and spend their lives becoming them all the while buying the lie that God isn't really God. In their altered mind state, He's just a little bit bigger sinner than they are and one day they will equal Him and overcome Him. These people constantly seek to discover themselves through becoming their careers, their marriages, their religions, their kids, their philosophies, and their things. They delight in quiz after quiz that expose their wonderful self and measure their IQ's relentlessly. They cherish their 'quirks', oftentimes pretending that God admires their sins and quirks too. After all, this is what makes them special and the amazing person that they are convinced that they are. Please realize that these quirks are not what they appear to be. All wrong thinking acted on is not of God. Where do you think it comes from? Where do you think the future of those who seek to establish another truth will end up at? Should you adore your quirks and your faults seeing that they do not originate from God's mind? How many people think they are gifted, special, talented, and amazing all on their own and they seek their counsel through psychics, mediums, and demonic friendships with a passion? Some even claim that they are special because they can easily communicate with the dead and the dead move through them to tell them of the spirit world. Where do you think these people will go? They are of their father the devil and many religious and spiritualist are already in Hades. I hope that you will not be so foolish. Salvation isn't a mystery. You simply go to be with the one you love.

For the vain and the proud, the bait is too much. They give in to the lie for love of self gain. Do you realize that self does not exist? God is all that there is and for all who try to create what cannot be you have wasted the time that God granted you to find Him. He is your true Self. All that you will ever discover outside of Him in you will be lies. There is nothing outside of Truth and to know any other way, thought, or emotion other than Him is to know death in your being. Your 'self', the one that spends hours trying to make itself amazing and godlike, is a myth, a lie, a devil. Should it not cease and desist, you will get to go dwell with all the lie lovers— forever.

I feel for those who learn how to contact and work with the dead. It is a stronger illusion of growing spiritually. Because a spirit knows little to no time restrictions or interferences in the demonic realm they travel by just thinking and can communicate instantly between people on opposite sides of the globe. People falsely assume that these powers are their own or that they control the spirits that they are using. This again, is part of the unclean spirits game. You think you are amazing and they help you to believe it! One person I came across bragged that they could talk to your spooks from anywhere and ask it(them) to leave. This is commonly done with those who practice spiritualism. This is not wise either and I suggest staying away from practices who do those things. Reiki is among the practices that one should avoid as well as any psychic or medium. You will only set up an e-mail account with a diseased soul. Not a good idea, okay? Your own spirit does have ability. These abilities are not to be confused with using other spirits. I remind everyone, that any action taken that does not originate from God in you is an action that should not be done. Meddling in other people's lives for self gain is wrong on any level. As long as you do what you do because it honestly helps someone else grow in truth and you do not seek to gain then you can do things like remote viewing, mind reading, and spirit interceptions. Make sure that your heart is in the right place before you even attempt to influence another soul. Otherwise there really can be 'hell' to pay. Contacting deceased people to ask curious questions is not of God and will cost you. Unclean spirits are diseased in frequency and will harm you.

Interestingly, unclean spirits usually hang around the things and people that they were emotionally attached to when they had a body of their own. Their lost loved ones are the ones they think of the most and for that reason they stay near family and usually on the father's side. Many don't want to leave the graveyards they are buried in. I believe that these respect God the most and are staying out of trouble, hoping for a better judgment day.

Did you ever notice how severely demon possessed the man in the tomb was that Jesus freed, you know, the one who lived near the graveyard? When Jesus set him free and he had collected a legion of unclean spirits. Graveyards and ghosts go together and people have known that for a long time. Those who are around the dead a lot are setting themselves up for disaster. If you are a mortician or mow grave yards, I pray that you set up a firewall against demonic spirits. You really need to know how to protect yourself by aligning your thoughts and emotions to HF and learn how to do a proper exorcism.

Unclean spirits are in essence energy. Because they operate on a low frequency they can chill a room. I am still uncertain if it is the amount of spirits that show up or the lowest frequency ones who are the ones detected. One can buy or make cameras that pick them up as well. I had one leave me with a strong electrical snap during a session of repentance once. Boy was I surprised! I was most definitely brought to attention. It is important to understand that they are to your body a 'negative' energy in that they remove the Life force in your spirit that keeps you well and all negative thoughts (thoughts that do not originate from God) will slowly bring death to your body.

Every person has unclean spirits coming and going on a regular basis. We must resist them when they enter so that they will flee. If you act upon their thoughts or ways, they have a legal reason to stay. After all, you are simply joining yourself to them, becoming at one with them; you are their compadre, their buddy and friend.

All people on earth have demonic entry as every single person on earth has some wrong thoughts that they move from. I often jokingly tell people to quit possessing the demons and leave them alone. Sin brings death to your body. You can see how it works and how simple it really is if you take religious rhetoric out of the picture.

It is kind of like a computer virus. They died of a virus and if they enter you, eventually you will receive the same virus and die too.

I conversed with a Catholic priest once who strongly opposed the doctrine of unclean spirits as the souls of humans. However, even he had to confess that he'd seen a healing after casting a deceased aunt out of a woman who had cancer. The

149

unclean spirit kept screaming at him, 'that's not my name' when he would call it the demon of cancer. It's kept screaming that it was the aunt that had died. The same cancer the aunt had was the exact same illness killing the woman who was being delivered. After expelling the demonic spirit, the woman was healed. How many healings would the church experience if they would just face the truth? Unclean spirits would face their worst nightmare! People would be healed in droves! Will they come into the Light?

Let me show you though, what a stronghold that unclean spirits have on people. This priest still refused to see the truth even though he'd witnessed it with his own eyes and continued to blaspheme God by saying I was speaking lies and misleading people. The forum also deleted all the threads with the information on it but left those made bearing titles like 'Stupid Old Testament'. People don't want to know where they are going without Christ and they want those who died to be 'well' no matter how they lived. They want to bury the dead and believe that they are just 'resting'. This false comfort is plan 'B' should plan 'A' not work out and somehow their twisted minds believe that if they don't admit the Truth it will go away. They already know they aren't living for the Truth but they love their lies so much that they would rather die in them than repent. And they will too. They don't want to see their own fate, a liar seldom does, and so they just look away and make up something that suits them, like Nephilims, fallen angels, and 40,000 religions or versions of the Truth. This is how to die, by the way, and come up with things like Evolution, the Darwin Theory, and the Big Bang Theory.

To be a follower of Truth, you have to be willing to see it at any cost. You can't live for your lusts and move out of self interest and come up with God. The further you are away from self, the clearer you will see. You must want Reality no matter how many friends it cost you, no matter how much money you lose, or how successful or unsuccessful you will be in this world's eyes. Your heart must be bent on knowing the way it 'really' is and doing what is 'really' right without regard to self or self interest.

The religious are the hardest to reach with the truth. The reason? They have hardened their heart the most against God. They looked at God's face and loved themselves instead whereas the sinner looks only at his own face. I have a saying that the Holy Spirit gave to me concerning the religious.

"Religion: Man discovering himself as god."

When you seek the Truth so it will serve you, you will never see or know the Truth. You moved from a low frequency thought and who is going to respond and bring you your answer? What you will discover is yourself as truth. When all that you do is centered on you, you become all that you know. Can you really save yourself? If you love yourself the most, you are soon to find out.

What are we really? Do we have the potential to be gods? If not, don't you think it is all a big waste of time? If you are really designed to function successfully in only one way, on only one frequency range, don't you think it futile to seek another? We are designed for a specific purpose, just like all of creation and can only be saved if we move in accordance to Him. God will bring about His purpose for creation and He isn't taking votes or directions from us on how to do it. He is Truth, the immovable unchangeable Rock. It is better to stand on the Rock then have the Rock fall on you.

Mankind has simply outsmarted himself. He has, like Satan, desired his own fantasy so bad, loving himself, adoring himself, and living for himself that he will end up losing Life completely if he doesn't see the Truth and desist. In the end all his lie loving will get him nothing but forever in an abyss.

Jesus, who was God incarnate, said he was not good. So just who do we think we are seeing that we are full of erroneous thoughts and ways? Do you see the arrogance in it all and why those who go out to seek glory and fame end up in Hades with their spirit and being in complete agony? We really are nothing of ourselves. It is the Truth! It is the honest to God Truth. People who live otherwise will die in their sins. 'You', the person who thinks he's

152

something, must die to live.

We live in perhaps the most Godless society since the days of creation. I write about Truth because I love Him, not because I think I will sell a lot of books. Writing about the Truth in today's world is definitely not a get rich quick scheme. If you've made it this far, you are most definitely able to bear some Truth.

Here is an example of how demons work. In voodoo if a person wishes to curse you they make a doll with your body's vibrational channels/frequencies on it. They use pieces of your hair or something and create a replica of your body's vibrations. Then they think of the most hateful thoughts that they can. This anger and extreme rage draws the most powerful demonic spirits to them. Once they feel the surge of energy they concentrate on the area of the doll picturing you. This is your spiritual e-mail address. The needle is then inserted into the doll and the spirits released to the doll or into your own spirit man. They have 'channeled' them to you. If they really hate you, they will destroy the doll by burning it or something of that nature. This sends the demonic spirits into action against your entire spirit man. Dark witches and those who work directly with demonic spirits are phishing the spiritual internet all the time. They take orders from the spirits and work in conjunction with them.

When we hate other people, think nasty mean

thoughts of them, we in essence are killing them by sending them spirits. This is why Jesus said that whosoever hates his brother without a cause is guilty of murder....because you are killing him....just slowly rather than all at once.

Wrong emotions, actions, thoughts, and ways draw devils to us. Direct communication with the dead can be a deadly fate. I am not going to tell you how to see demons on your own face and on the face of others, I do not want to give you more information than necessary but I want you to know that anyone can see the unclean spirits that infiltrate their lives. This information is taught in my seminars in a safe setting and only used in deliverances. Young people like to fool with unclean spirits and are curious by nature and in this case it isn't a good thing. Remember, evil spirits are the main reason that people are sick and dying. You don't want to call them to you and have a séance and enjoy their presence. They speak mainly and mostly lies and have missed heaven's door, so why would you want their wisdom? You cannot become powerful as God has all power, so why be a fool and let a demonic spirit kill, steal, and destroy your life? Why join the delusional? Who is the fool then? The proud are the most foolish people on earth.

There is a pathway to God. Demons try to keep you from it. They come to steal it away from you should you actually find it. It is our own wicked hearts that keep us from seeing or seeking this sacred path and also that which causes us to fall from it.

8 And an highway shall be there, and a way, and it shall be called The way of holiness; the unclean shall not pass over it; but it *shall be* for those: the wayfaring men, though fools, shall not err *therein*.

Isaiah 35:7-9 (KJV)

There is a way/frequency to heaven. I wonder how many will actually find it. Think of all the wasted lives, all the people trying to be 'something' that die in the process. How many times has this world repeated its success theory of money, fame, fortune, and glory apart from God only to rot in the ground and roam the earth as a vagabond.

Do you realize that if you talk yourself into believing a lie, living for that lie, and then dying in the lie that all you've done is close your eyes to the Truth and successfully died to life itself? Your accomplishment in the earth is that you just destroyed yourself....congratulations. This is how lives are wasted every day.

Demons see our faults and love that we love them. They capitalize on them, exploit them, and we stand there just scratching our heads as if we've been ambushed. If we weren't so in love with our faults and our demons, we might actually be able to escape.

1 Awake, awake; put on thy strength, O Zion; put on thy beautiful garments, O Jerusalem, the holy city: for henceforth there shall no more come into thee the uncircumcised and the unclean. 2 Shake thyself from the dust; arise, *and* sit down, O Jerusalem: loose thyself from the bands of thy neck, O captive daughter of Zion.

Isaiah 52:1-2 (KJV)

Shake the 'dust' off of you. The demonic spirits that weigh you down, the lie lovers that come to woo you, hoping to gainsay the truth. Instead of giving them your ear, your heart, and your mind, being a faithful little repeater station of low frequency, why don't you come into reality, the truth of your faults and the ways in and around you that are not correct. Stop being afraid to see that you are not perfect and that you need God. It should be your desire that from henceforth no LF thoughts will come from your spirit. Loose yourself from their bonds, their lies of prosperity, fame, fortune, and power. O captive daughter of Zion, you are captive because you sold yourself into it. You loved Egypt with all its fake wonderful finery, worship of people, and self righteous lifestyles. The tombs of the dead, the belief in the continuation of a corrupt life, this is what the Egyptians loved and you envy their lie. They loved and adored themselves and you want to do the same. What is the fate of those who love lies? Where will they go? All who emit low frequencies will one day be gone. Tuned out by the Creator as vile and corrupt.

2 And it shall come to pass in that day, saith the LORD of hosts, *that* I will cut off the names of the idols out of the land, and they shall no more be remembered: and also I will cause the prophets and the unclean spirit to pass out of the land.

Zech 13:2 (KJV)

Again, *all* spirits who are unclean will one day pass from this land. They will forever be in torment for having turned a deaf ear to the Truth in their lives. They saw the Truth and wanted the lie. I pray that you and I are not among that number and that we will be the humble and contrite and willing to see our faults; to know the difference between right and wrong and choose only right in our hearts.

Seven

Your Spirit

The essence of Spirit and spirituality....

How important is it to you to discern where you are coming from seeing that where you come from determines where you are going? Do you realize that we have been killing God/Life in us? By shutting down the Conscience in our life we have shut down God.

If people don't put Truth first place in their hearts and seek Him with all of their heart, mind, and soul, how can they really be of God? God is Spirit and Truth how can you be of Him if you don't like the Truth? He is the All-Spirit God. How can you serve Him if you move from a carnal demonic mind set and live for a physical world and just do church and world activities and then be in unison with the all Spirit God? One is either moving from 'Spirit and Truth' or 'spirit and lies'. For all who live only by the evidence of the physical world and according to it accepting only that which they 'choose' to see, they will live a life of lies and deception.

All who love the dark cannot love the Light for if they did, they would come to the Light. The Light created the darkness, just as you create a shadow. God's Spirit is all and in all. Remember, God's Spirit overrides, rules, creates, and is all matter. God is perfect vibrations and we must become perfect like Him to be with Him.

Everything that your spirit is experiencing in frequencies will soon be shouted to the world by your body.

2 For there is nothing covered, that shall not be revealed; neither hid, that shall not be known.
Luke 12:2 (KJV)

The point here, that I want you to deeply grasp, is that the spiritual world is not subject to the physical, but the physical subject to the spiritual. Everyone will soon see who you are as your flesh will tell the story. This is why disease, famine, death, and wars will never cease until the spirits behind them are gone. We cannot 'save the planet' when that which is destroying it is still present and nearly untouched.

Even the medical realm recognizes healings and will often tell their patients to seek the Lord for help when they cannot help them themselves. Many doctors also refuse to operate on a depressed person. Why? What difference should it make if a person is just like a car, physical, and needing a few spare parts? It is well known that a depressed person can die easily in surgery and so many doctors will not operate on you in a state of depression. Why? Your life source/HF are diminished and they know you won't heal well.

In the physical world we understand that power means force. Water falling and hitting a wheel for instance can do everything from grinding flour to generating electricity, depending on what we do with it. If we take this same basic principal to the spiritual realm of cause and effect you will see that it applies there as well. Spirit is the causation and the physical world becomes the effect and God is all Energy. All sin/wrong thinking acted on will lead to death. All truth/correct understanding leads to Life.

God made your spirit. The energy is His. He built you a body and put your spirit in it and created your soul. They aren't yours. All that you are is His to do with as He pleases. Never forget this. Live in great respect of your Creator and be wise, choose life.

You don't own anything. We live like we do and then we die deceived and angry. When the body He blessed you with expires, if you did not find the truth in your heart, you return to the void from whence you came. Your spirit and soul are His and it will be up to Him to do with it as He chooses, not you. Where does God send your spirit? What will He do with you? Shouldn't we live in fear and respect of His Truth and His ways? If He, who does not lie, says that sin will kill you, shouldn't we listen? If he puts laws into place that govern the spiritual world wouldn't it behoove man to pay heed?

Everyone consciously knows that they will die. Most of us pretend it won't happen, ignoring the plethora of graveyards, and due to its depressing aspect, we push it out of our minds and pad ourselves with medical plans and insurances; as if they would stay our execution. However, the massive amount of burial plots and booming business of the funeral homes would attest to the failure of our plans and efforts to remain immortal.

I have had the blessed experience to feel my spirit body separate from my physical body. It was sort of caught between the two worlds. In the spirit world, it felt like a body, but in this world it felt like a floating balloon! To say I completely understand the worlds would be a farce, but I do know that they are both there and somehow overlap.

A spiritual body feels much like a physical body in the spiritual realm. You can feel your extremities and the bodies of others but there is a cold dark feeling present. You immediately realize that the sun is not shinning and there's no sensation of bodily warmth that we are use to or a grounding sensation. Instead there is a light feeling and a sense of not being tied down and a sort of buoyant sensation. I felt light, cold and empty, my spiritual cord obviously was not severed.

Having this experience has really helped me comprehend how spirits move and what they feel and feel like. They are already in so much darkness and that world is so cold that it is no wonder that they seek bodies to dwell in for warmth. Being a spirit was in a sense freeing in that one did not have the weight of the flesh or the limitations that flesh has, but you didn't 'radiate' either or have a sense of warmth or belonging.

I've also felt the 'claws' of demons on my spirit so I know that spirits can hurt each other. I was 16 at the time when that occurred and it is a common experience amongst those suffering from deep depression. I know of several others in my own family who experienced the same thing. Some people will wake up with bite marks or claw marks on their bodies. I was in the mode between asleep and awake and tormented like that on several occasions. Like I said, this is a common experience for those who have strong demonic encounters. Demons can chew, claw, and tear another spirit and it often is revealed on the flesh as a flesh wound. They are pulling at your vibrations and attacking you. This would also prove that spirit affects matter as many who waken from being clawed in their sleep find the marks on their bodies upon awakening. Spirits do feel pain and can inflict it as well. So if you think dying will stop your pain, think again! Suicide is not the answer and end to your pain but the beginning of more misery.

I mentioned before that spirits that are not bound to a body and do not seem to know much of a time lapse when traveling. They can be almost immediately where ever they think and they can give and receive information just as fast. We do not realize that we have some use of those functions before crossing over and laugh and are amazed at all our 'coincidences'. For example, you think of someone and the next thing you know that person is calling you.

"Wow," you say, "I was just thinking about you!", amazed by the weird coincidence, when in truth you sent them a message first and called them causing them to call you. Some people will receive the message, think of you in return and then you call them instead! We don't realize how we all have spiritual abilities as we have spirits and telepathy is just a function of our spirit, not an occult action. I find it interesting that so many religious people scowl at anything remotely spiritual and call it 'cultish' or assign it to witchcraft and then promptly use it without realizing it in their own every day life. Your spirit also can sense someone's auras and spiritual energy. This is why you can instantly like or dislike someone. Your spirit already reads theirs. It just depends on how 'tuned in' you are as to how much and what you hear. Your first impressions are almost always correct because they have not been clouded yet by your thinking. Just what abilities does your spirit have? The bible says you are a new 'creature' in Christ Jesus....so what can that creature do? The word of knowledge is a gift whereby you can read someone's frequencies. You can tell where they are sinning and you are given immediate information on their life for their benefit.

Women are better at following their intuition and feelings due to the easier access to both sides of their brain. They are naturally more spiritual. Guys know this and it bugs them to no end......hence the overpopulation of female witches. The function of both sides of the brain, coupled with the innate gift of 'reading' spirits and others appears to give women an edge, but a Godly man, a man who truly puts God first, will go long and far as the bible attests. They don't stray as easy as women tend to. However, man's pride costs him years off of his life in worry and without ample sex to ease them, they die faster. I'm not suggesting that you women should go out and save your hubbies with sex, okay? This is merely an observation on spiritual conditions which is only cured in Christ. Women are more wishy washy which is what Paul was worried about. They tend to channel so easy that who knows what they are picking up and for this reason I suggest being neither male nor female. You really are neither in Christ. Begin to leave the flesh behind and become at one in Christ. There is no condemnation to those who are in Him and you can do all things in and of Him when you leave the flesh behind.

If people could only grasp the energies behind the scene they would change the way they view life and themselves. You are not your body, your body is in you. Every problem that you think is outside of you must affect you inwardly first. Watch out for 'falling in love' it is a sure sign that demons are in charge.

I was watching a TV. show awhile back. It was a famous show where people show the cool old house they bought and the history behind it. A woman on the show was just astounded at the 'coincidence' in her life. She fell in love with a house and bought it. Then she painstakingly went out and very selectively bought all the furniture her heart led her to buy and she placed it exactly where she thought 'she' liked it. Then to her surprise she found out the house had belonged to an aunt she had never met who had recently passed away. Afterwords she discovered an old photograph of the house and again was 'amazed' that she had not only bought every piece of identical furniture in the picture but she placed it all in the same setting in the house. Coincidence? Or was she getting help? Who is 'helping' you in your life?

To say that the spirit world is far away from our world is to live with one's head intentionally in the sand. Paul said that we don't wrestle against flesh and blood but against principalities and powers of the air. He is saying that it isn't your career, the flesh body you live in, the dog, the economy, or anything exterior to your being that is your problem. He said that the war was within.

23 But I see another law in my members, warring against the law of my mind, and

**bringing me into captivity to the law of sin which
is in my members.**

Romans 7:23 (KJV)

It isn't as if I need to tell you this. You and I both
know that the struggles come from within. We
understand that conflict as we live it every day. Like
the insects that lay larvae in an apple, we find our
enemy alive within us, growing, and ripping us
apart from the inside out. We can feel it. Everything
outside of us becomes an aggravation and extension
of the inward war; the constant gnawing and
devouring of what is precious to us. We understand
subconsciously that we war not against the tax
dollar, the latest communist regime, global
warming, our spouse, or the economy. These things
our heart knows. Our war is in spirit and can only be
fought in spirit. Woe to those who say the enemy is
not there or those who make it all about the
physical! How easy would it be for you if you were
invisible to destroy someone, especially if you could
get inside their mind and their feelings? See why the
world is sick? Our enemy has been going around in
stealth protecting its secret with a vengeance and
like the larvae, eating away at the heart of mankind;
pulling our spirits into the dust where they live.

The importance of this chapter is that I want you
to understand that the death of your body is not
what demons say that it is. Your problems are not
exterior to you, they are in you. You will not be

'released' to ascend to the light if you live in the
darkness. If you kill yourself, that's murder. Guess
where they don't get to go? One of the biggest lies
that evil spirits don't want you to know is that you
are not ascending in your own power. They believe
they are and so they preach this to you. There is no
goodness outside of God. The only salvation of
mankind is through God; who is Truth. To think that
'you' are ascending by your power and your
goodness is no different then Satan 'ascending' in all
his fake power and his fake goodness. You are not
god and cannot ascend upon any righteousness of
yourself...there isn't any outside of God. So to go
around and spend your life establishing what cannot
be is how to waste your life.

Look at many of the modern Christians. They
believe in themselves, not God. Have you actually
listened to their worship music? It isn't about God. It
is all about them. They stand for hours, hands lifted
high, adoring themselves. They believe that they are
good. They fully believe in themselves. They are
everything from gay, to extremely proud, hateful
and self righteous men-pleasers and they call it
'God'.

Many so called Christians are very in love with
themselves and in reality there is not much
difference between them and Satan. Those who love
themselves cannot know the truth and will not be
with God for they deny Him by simply believing in
themselves.

The church has a scheme. I will expound heavily

upon it in my ministry in hopes of setting people free. You are being brainwashed, fully fleeced, and left for dead. There is a great effort by the big evangelists and churches to keep you dead and in your fake salvation. Should you awaken, they would lose their money, their fame, and their glory which they are enjoying at your expense. I would love to see the Pharisees fail in their effort to destroy lives. I would love to see the huge churches become empty buildings as God's children leave behind the lies to become truly spiritual, walking their streets, and living and talking of Truth! You were never meant to serve a religion. You can feel it destroying you, but you know not where to turn. You are shamed into 'congregating' and 'becoming' them. May this book encourage you to break free and may you be blessed to escape religion to live unto Truth.

Evil spirits want you to believe you are good/god because they believe the same thing, that they are god too. One day, they think they will destroy God and take the throne. They will keep ascending up and up until one day the become Him. They've been trying it for years. They thought they killed God when they killed Jesus, but they were gravely mistaken.

Death to the physical body has been measured. That is to say that the spirit has 'weight' and an aura surrounding a person perishes upon death or sometimes a week before hand. Some people have seen strings of white wispy ghosts leave them right before their own spirit momentarily did. This is a pretty common experience with those who die and come back to life.

Often upon death a person is visited by a loved one. The bible says that the angels will come and get the saved, not a loved one. The fact that a person is seeing a loved one is not a good sign. It means that the person dying is probably not saved. I know of one person who even spoke in the voice of their dead husband and carried a full conversation with them audibly in themselves before death. This person was not saved and did not make it to heaven but went with her late husband having had full conversations in both voices weeks before she died. This was my grandmother.

When I do exorcisms I see their *human* faces in full color. The Holy Spirit tells me their names, I get histories, and full color pictures like the vehicle they were driving before they crashed or the death scene! I know, that I know, that I know, that unclean spirits are the spirits of the deceased. That is why some unclean spirits are smart, some are stupid, and they have human characteristics as many ministers have noticed. They have all the characteristics of a person.....because they are former people. People who died without God.

All spirits return to God to do with as He pleases. He denies unclean ones entry to heaven because they do not bow to Him nor confess His name and nor do they serve Him. He is Truth and no lies dwell with Him. They have no place in Truth.

Derik Prince said in his book 'And They Shall

Expel Demons' and I quote, "*It is hard for us to entertain the idea of a person without a body. Nevertheless, even though demons have not bodies, they have all the normally accepted marks of personality*".

Ministers know in their hearts who demons are, but if they confess what they know many Christians would not listen to them anymore, so rather than lose their ministries, their money, or the fame they lust after, they continue on with the lie.

I believe that Derik Prince honestly did not know who they were but was very close to discovering it for himself. Derik goes on the explain how demons would scream, "that's not my name!" when he would cast them out, calling them by their affliction while they spouted human names. He says on page 95 that he *"never had an impression that he was dealing with angelic beings"* and that they are earthbound creatures who bear all the marks of people. His summary is ended by saying that they are like people and not angelic type beings and that they are far too ignorant to be fallen angels. He almost found out the truth too bad religion blinded his eyes.

Eight

The Exorcist:

Qualities, strengths, and weaknesses

I've witnessed a lot of hype concerning exorcisms. If you've taken any time to look at it on the internet it will astound you. I've found people casting out things like the demon of deodorant, gay demons, demons in candles, dolls, you name it— it 'has' a demon! Everywhere you look there's an expert looney teaching the art of deliverance.

It occurred to me that this is just another way unclean spirits keep their real cover. It gives real deliverance a bad name like the weather balloon theory of Area 51. People are getting hurt for the games that are being played concerning deliverance. I also noticed that this particular area of ministry tends to attract the arrogant. It appears that the idea of being completely proud jerk and overpowering other jerks is more than some religious folks can endure and so they seek to 'become' amazingly awesome powerful spiritual unstoppable dynamic warriors. Meanwhile, all those who really need deliverance get destroyed for lack of real assistance.

Then, there are those who would be good at deliverance except that they make it all about themselves and money. Everything is the demon's fault and they are there to save the world. This theology gets old after awhile because everyone knows deep inside that it is their own sin that has them whipped and if they would 'resist' the devil they would be free 99 percent of the time. To live within the theology that 'the demon made me do it' is to live in denial of God Himself. Pride again is to blame as it refuses to repent because it would have to change.

There are no 'perfect' exorcists, only a perfect God working through imperfect man. I will say this, that the less sin that you have in you the stronger the exorcism. Even the Muslims know this. What does that say about Christiandom when the Muslims know more than most Christians on this subject? I want to make it clear here that God is no respecter of persons. You might have won the Nobel peace prize or a trophy of some kind but He really doesn't care nor will it sway His view of your sins that you practice. He is looking at your heart, not what you've told yourself is true about your own self. God's eyes are not dim. He is never conned and He sees you 'just' as you are.

An exorcist is nothing without God and so I'm not impressed by people's bragging or boasting. All glory 'is' God's, all power is His, and glory 'belongs' to Him. Which means that we don't have any. All power, wisdom, love, and peace belong to the Father of Lights with whom there is no variable neither shadow of turning. He is pureness. Not one drop of truth is outside of Him. Not one drop of lies is within Him. All existence is within Him and nothing was made without Him.

The stronger you know Him, the more of Him that will flow through you. This is what displaces the spirits of this world. God flowing through you, angels moving on God's words coming out of your mouth, spoken by Him in you. There are no 'shortcuts' to Truth. You cannot run out and get what you need at the last minute. It takes time to get to know Him, time to let go of the sin and false thinking you were taught in this world. It is the oil in your lamp that cannot be gotten in a moments notice. Don't waste your life. Don't spend your spare time chasing shadows, lies, and fairy tales of self. Seek the Truth. Seek His face. Honestly try to know Him, His character, His ways, and His heart. Don't seek your television set, smut magazines, prideful ambitions, money and the world and church leadership positions—you will lose your soul. Feed your soul the Truth(higher frequencies) and reap life into your being.

I am not going to cover the exorcism process in this book. It is taught at my conferences because you need hands on experience and you need to be able to ask questions and get immediate answers. If you want to be an exorcist, it is a noble thing to do for the Lord and others. I learn more everyday and hope to bless others in all that I know for those who have the heart for it. I also don't consider myself in the running for 'best exorcist in the world'.

One thing that I learned from ministry so far is that I don't have a big enough heart. An exorcist must have a heart the size of Montana! You have to be willing to go the extra mile and be willing to be disliked for doing it, humiliated if nothing happens, and able to not get puffed up when something amazing does happen. You must have it settled in your heart that your reward comes from God alone and be willing to be alone a lot. I simply am not there yet. I can feel it, see it, and God is working on me but I can tell that it comes from many days of spending time with the Father.

The deliverance process cannot be about yourself. You have to be able to lay yourself aside and follow the Holy Spirit. If you make someone's exorcism about you, you will hurt the person you are trying to help. You risk attaching the person to you through abuse. Again, this is the essence and foundation of brainwashing. If you see that someone is trying to prove something to you or making their own exorcism about you or them the exorcism should be called off. Why? You cannot move from a low frequency thought/flesh and do God's work. He will not bless the exorcism and the outcome will be twisted.

Also, as an exorcist, don't expect to be well liked. Demons pick up right away that you are more than able to dispose of them and so you must expect them to act up in people, especially family, and be willing to overlook it as they all will most likely abandon you and/or attack you. If you've given your life to God, this won't really bother you, but if you are existing and living through others this will hurt and possibly destroy you.

The purer your heart, the stronger the exorcism and more peaceful your walk. Realize that everything you do is not up to you. You are on God's guidance system now. He has the controls, knows what's best, and is in charge. You are not your own. Self really must die in order to do this in a real way.

Block out the world, what others think of you, and just go forward. Life isn't about you anymore, you died. Put yourself in that grave and don't get up. If God requires you to let go of family, do it. If God takes away a dream, let it go. He knows better than you....just let Him lead you all the way. Be willing to trust what you can't see because He asks it of you and you know that He is right no matter what you can or can't see. Be willing to live underneath the feet of someone who hates you without hating them back. It is your job. Do it heartily unto the Lord and know that your reward comes from heaven, not people. This will keep your head clear.

Sometimes when the clouds seem dark and I feel

the crying and emptiness of my spirit needing His Light and Love, I just close my eyes and curl up and envision me in the palm of His cupped hand. Sometimes He covers me with His other one. I can feel His warm energy covering me. It will wash me from head to toe and back and forth, hugging me. This keeps me focused on His comfort, rather than the situation and emotions of fear or doubt that are trying to get in. Rest in Him and He will give you the wisdom, warmth, and energy you need. I sometimes quote pure scriptures as I fall to sleep. You know, the ones that He has already enlightened to your understanding. This guides, protects, and nourishes my heart.

Often, by morning, the solution to the problems I was facing will have arrived during the night. Whatever it was that nearly beset me subsided in the dark of night and I am able to go forward, rested and calm. I have found that it is better to be still in Him then busy in me. Busy minds make for the devil's work shop. What can't the devils produce in a mind that seeks a way apart from Truth?

Every person in Christ is supposed to be an exorcist. It is part of the great commission but I believe that some are called in a deeper way. Don't let the title puff you up. It is another trick of the demon to get you to move from pride so you are ineffective. Know that power and success is all in God's hands, not yours. You are not some elite force and the only spiritual Christian out there, okay?

Don't let the 'aspect' of this job go to your head. It will be His Spirit that casts out the demon and heals the sick, not yours. See the truth in it and don't pull the weight of it upon your own shoulders. God has His reasons for everything He does and they are all 'correct' whether we see them or not. Learn to trust Him in a simple way. Don't over complicate it or make it about you.

I like to have time to seek God's face before any exorcism. Often God will give me the name of the demon or tell me of the person's situation coming for help or let me know not to do it. Sometimes I will see the face of the unclean spirit causing the trouble. I like to have the time to purify and examine my own heart so that I can help in the most effective way possible. Never be hasty when you lay hands on someone. They may have tons of unrepentant sin in their lives that God is in the process of dealing with them on. Do not partake of anything that you have no peace in. Peace **is** God's approval. No peace....no approval.....it is that simple.

It is foolish to limit God. All the creation powers are in you when the Holy Spirit is present. It is the same Spirit that hovered over the waters and created the whole earth. What can't he do? All the diseases and demons in the world can't stand against Him. Just make sure you are moving with Him. You can easily grow out bones, destroy any illness, and send any demon high tailing it in the other direction. It occurred to me the other day that if a bone can grow out a limb should be just as easy. What can't God do? Dear God, give us the faith that we need!

Patience is the mark of a mature soul. This has been a lesson that has not come easy for me. I think I was born for the microwave generation. I simply don't see the point in waiting most of the time and have had a lot to learn concerning it. Patience is huge when it comes to doing God's work. You cannot have your own agenda or time table. God's work is always done His way and in His time...Every Time.

I want you to think about your ministry. Everyone has a ministry. Your life is your ministry. How are you doing it? Are you a grumpy, angry, short fused mommy? Are you a dad who has no time for his kids? Are you impatient at work and complain? How is your ministry performed? Are you honest? Will God be able to say, "well done...thou good and faithful (to what you knew was right) or will he say depart from me you who practice sin(wrong thinking.)"

Were we faithful to what we knew was right? God is truth, love, peace, honesty, kindness, sincerity, all that is good and true....are we faithful to what we know is right? Or are we supporting what is wrong in us?

Every exorcism should be based on doing what you know is right not from some hidden agenda such as to make a name for yourself or get ahead in ministry or to impress anyone or for money. Your motives need to be pure. Your life, the way you live, will determine how effective of an exorcist you are.

Who is called to be an exorcist? All who are truly saved will have this sign following them.

17 And these signs shall follow them that believe; In my name shall they cast out devils; they shall speak with new tongues;

18 They shall take up serpents; and if they drink any deadly thing, it shall not hurt them; they shall lay hands on the sick, and they shall recover.
Mark 16:17-18 (KJV)

This is how you know that you are His. These signs will follow you. If they aren't, you should find out why because it means your faith is broken. This is a description of what God looks like in the earth, moving. He casts out demons, heals the sick, and poison things don't hurt Him, and He speaks in Spirit, moves in Spirit and is the 'all' Spirit God.

When people move with Him, this how they will look too and if He is in you, these things will happen. You will speak in tongues, you will heal the sick, cast out demons, be able to take deadly poison into your system and it will not hurt you. That means you aren't a health nut, seeking to save yourself from every preservative and afraid for your well being, running from fear, eating or not eating from fear, and living from fear.

Sick people will recover because your spiritual energy will simply restore theirs. It isn't some mystery. It is a scientific fact and you won't be thinking about this world's version of health care as your alternative to God either. All you need comes from your Father's hand. You only have one God.

When you see that people choose to think wrong thoughts and intentionally love them and you see that you honestly don't need a single thing from them then your fears will diminishes to the proportion of revelation you receive. It is not hard to walk quietly with God if you are really hearing from Him. It is impossible if you are pretending to hear Him.

If you are really attached to someone you will see it is because you are using that person in some form or another. Most attachments are brought on through abuse or lust. That attachment is detrimental to you both. It may be that you need to see yourself as a good person so you can feel good about yourself or that you are always a 'victim' and in a crisis. Living like this allows you to stay continually focused on your own poor soul and enables you to justify worshiping your own self. The mind set behind abuse is one that always sees itself as getting shafted by a horrible person who cruelly takes advantage of your good soul.

180

Arrogance is key in the mind of a victim. If you live off the energy of another person it means that you are a user. You need a revelation(s) to get free. Don't despair, seek God and He will show you the way.

Pride in us does foolish things and like David said, "cleanse thou me from my secret faults"— everyone has them. Your hearts aim must be to get rid of faults by honest desire to be closer to God. The more faults you have, the more demons can enter you during exorcisms and every day life.

To be strong in faith you need deep revelations on Truth/God/Reality in your soul. You cannot go around with your concocted version of reality, the latest theologians version of scripture, or such, and be at one with God. You cannot be holding up your ego like a lamp in front of you and letting it lead your way and then expect to find God at the end of your egotistical path.

Many people live for themselves and some do it in God's name. They worship themselves in His name and call themselves good, pat themselves on the back, and aspire to take the throne and wear the crown. In their twisted little minds, God is just there to serve them and they see themselves above His Word; spouting scriptures and waving bibles as if it were God Himself on their side doing their bidding. They hate you in God's name. It's amazing how they think that God approves of all their hate and sin.

If you follow the Truth you'd better not be concerned about popularity. Don't place your heart on people and put anyone on a pedestal. People just trip up and fall, even you do, so don't put the pressure on them to be 'God' in your life. Idolatry is as wrong now as it was when Moses held the tablets of stone. How many Christians do you know that worship 'important' ministers? Did you know that there is no such thing anyway? It is a plastic title worn by deceived souls. People only worship others because they wish to be like them. Idolatry is a condition of the heart and for those who aspire to have their own pedestal your fruit is hanging for all to see.

The old saying, "birds of a feather flock together" is true. Those who love their sin will find more sin lovers like themselves to ease their guilt of sin loving. You see it all the time. If that isn't ugly enough, then they use God's name to back it up thinking that you certainly have to agree with them now because they have God on their side and He taught them all the hypocrisy that they know. They only fool those who believe and practice the same lie they love. All glory hounds live at the same dog ranch.

What kind of people do you associate and feel closeness to? An honest observation will go a long way in getting close to God.

Demons don't want you to know that they are there. They like you to think I am wrong about them. They will push you to do so. They don't want you to know that they are in people, moving and working and ruining lives. They want you to believe in yourself; your wonderful, awesome, amazing fake phoney non-existent self. They want you to go to church and feel good about 'you' and seek to be special and okay. They love it when you tithe and lead you to think that that makes up for the sin in your heart. Did you try to buy Jesus with silver this month?

Demonic spirits encourage you to believe that you are a 'good' person so you will never truly repent. They like it when you say stern religious things, quote scripture, go to church, and don't mean a bit of it. Hey, they are hypocrites too! As long as people think you're good, you're happy because you get to keep on sinning and others love you a lot cause you're just like them. Demons love it that you are happy in your sin, cause they are happy in your sin too. They can do whatever they want with you as long as they live within your boundaries and areas of deception. You find your thrills in deceiving others and yourself and in such you will never know God. I hope that you are not like that, I really do.

The time is coming when no man can talk of the things of heaven. This world will not tolerate any form of Truth. It will be in its final stages of deception to usher in the one world government and the ideologies that come with it. If you are one of the few who are able to endure sound thoughts and concepts, don't let the abounding wickedness get to you. Have you ever deep cleaned a room?

Everything gets pulled apart and sorted out and the room is a disaster! You toss, sort, and reorganize and the room is restored to wellness. So it is in these end times. The world is a big mess. God is cleaning up things and reconciling mankind back to Himself in His time, His way. All people will and do answer to Him. They don't have a choice. Don't worry about making everyone do the right thing in your life. It's God's life now and He'll take care of all of it. God will do it all. All you have to do is love and obey Him. See how simple it really is?

You will find that people who love themselves supremely will get tired of you quite quickly when you don't play their foolish games. There's no need for harsh words, mocking, or criticism. All who do evil will reap evil. It is a spiritual law that applies to you too. So remember, evil has its rewards. Be fearful and respectful and shrink back from all that your heart shows you in that regards.

Don't beat yourself up for mistakes. God is bigger than your mistakes. See them, feel the ugly truth of it with remorse, wish in your heart to get past them and let God deal with them. Don't hide from them and pretend they aren't there. Demons live within deception. The more honest you are, the less they can do to you and with you. Just watch yourself, quit looking away, and the faults will soon go away. Hide from them and they are sure to stay. Humility is the key to a close relationship with the Truth.

If you are a prideful person it just means that you don't know God very well. The Truth is extremely humbling. If you are the kind of person that gets angry when you are told your faults then you are not humble. You should know your faults and be well aware of your misgivings and in repentance of them; seeking to rise above them by revelations from your Father.

Spending time with God is not what most folks make it out to be. They poise themselves in a proper manner, perhaps one hand in the air, the eyes closed and they breathe in and feel their own wondrous righteousness. You might as well have blown your nose and called it a day. Foolish child, God can see your arrogant soul. Stop the games and go somewhere in a secret place where you can come off your pride and have a man to man talk with the Truth. Start fessing up to your sins!

True worship isn't when you sing hymns in harmony dressed in matching robes or make tears to come down your cheeks as you worship your lofty ideals. True worship is when your soul lauds and invites the Truth within its spirit and thanks God for showing it to you.

Demons don't want that to happen and would rather you play church all day long seven days a week in matching choir robes, fancy buildings, and give you many famous pastors. They'll fund your buildings, build your programs, and help you bake the pie for the pastor but just try and sit down in

God's presence and be honest and see what comes of it?

One woman I knew had three cd players burned out by demons as she tried to play the meditation cds that I sent her. Yet the demons had no problem with her going to church.

I double dare you to be honest with yourself. Just how ugly are you? How many demons are in 'your' closet? Can you even tell me your faults? Can you even tell you your faults?

People love pointing out each others faults. That way, they don't have to think about their own and can justify their own sins according to the sins of others. What happens to you when you measure yourself by a failing grade? Instead of having God's Spirit to be our guide we look at another person who may be missing the mark entirely and we go by what they are doing or saying and live 'better' than them, as if it made us a good person. This will bring spiritual disaster. Never do that. Let that person be like an alien from another planet. If they think that salvation consists of going to church on certain days, wearing only black, taking their watch off during church, putting on special hats, gathering naked under a fig tree or whatever their crazy beliefs are, look at them as alien beings from another planet and get your heart set on pleasing only the Father. Leave people alone in their walks with God and only participate where God leads you to. People-pleasers are miserable people. Idolatry has a price.

Let your yes be yes and your no be no, in other words, be set in what you know is right and wrong. You make a mistake, see it, feel it, and acknowledge the Truth in all you do and let what He shows you light the pathway before your feet. Stay humble and small so He can be great in you. I know that this isn't what most religious people are pushing nowadays but I'm telling you that the more you try to be God the more miserable you will become. Mistakes are how you discover the 'right' way to go. Don't let a mistake stop you from seeking God. Let it be your beginning.

I know this may not seem relevant here, but I often take really, really hot baths. There are times when you just need a 'do over'. Wash it all away and repent and ask God to help and get back on that horse of Truth and Justice and Wisdom and don't let go of her. When you fall, don't hide it, don't run, and don't lie. Just suck in your pride...you made the mistake, own up to it.....cry some real tears of repentance if they come and God will strengthen you to continue the race you are on and ask God for the wisdom to destroy the reason you fell. His word promises that He will give it to you liberally and not criticize you.

You will find that God knows your faults and you much better than you do. Trust His lead in your life. Stop questioning Him on every detail as if He has to answer to you. Be respectful. If you don't understand something then ask for wisdom. He gives it liberally to those who ask and I have found this to be more than true. With pure wisdom you can overcome anything. Don't let a situation daunt or destroy you. God has overcome this world and He is in you.

The real strength of the exorcist is in the ability to be humble and truly spiritual. You can tell if you are in accordance with God by your emotions. What does the heart of God feel? Is He hateful, arrogant, prideful, nasty, greedy, mean, cruel, selfish, does He enjoy the pain of others, does He get a kick out of hurting someone? What emotion is behind what you are about to do? If you only move from what you want or according to your flesh how can you do God's work? You can't. You will do your work, dead, ugly, stinking works. The angels will not uphold what you say and you will die in your sins and everything you do will be accomplished in a corrupt manner.

When we war against the evil spirit world, the corrupt thoughts and ways, we cannot find our strength from the physical world because it is just an extension of corruption. This war in us, this battlefield of the mind, is called and referred to by Paul as flesh. We know that real flesh cannot war as a dead body cannot cause any problems to the living? This war is one of high and low frequency.....right and wrong, good and evil. It is that sinful nature in you, namely spirits working in conjunction with your own wrong thoughts....this is your flesh.

I have discovered, to my wondrous delight, that if you remove the demon's ways and you honestly repent and change, the demon spirit is evicted— permanently! We change frequency in our spiritual energy when we align with God's energy and the lower frequencies are abandoned and demons are not able to enter or use one. It is amazing. One unclean spirit left with an electrical discharge! Outstanding!

This is why Jesus was able to heal by touch and why we are supposed to lay hands on the sick. We are supposed to be full of this same Positive Energy. Instead, the majority of ministers pass on their demonic spirits or dark energy as they live in sin and preach from the flesh. Be very careful who you have pray for you as you may get more than you bargained for.

It is my hope that the church, the real children of Truth, will come into the knowledge of who demons are and what these spirits are doing to them. Even if they jangle on how to deal with them, I wish they could at least get the understanding of who the enemy really is. It is hard to watch them suffer, die, and cry out and follow the demons to their doctors and then watch the doctors help them straight on to the grave. I wish I could at least tell them who is behind the scene in their lives destroying it.

If you are able to accept and hear what I am

saying know that at this point and time you are a minority. Most hear me and some accept it at first, then in a few days the demons freak them out and I either never hear from them again or they align themselves against me with great vigor thinking that if they make me go away, so will the Truth.

One pastor I know was immediately struck with fear. He took it upon himself to make some ugly fliers up and sent them to every church nearby to let them know that I was evil. It is amazing. The demons in that pastor didn't seem to see the local churches as threats at all nor did they send fliers out warning against the nearby openly practicing wiccan church. Who are demons really afraid of and who are they trying to protect?

It was weird because not only did I have pastors sending out hate mail but I had witches sacrificing cats and putting curses on me, now tell me why were the witches and the pastors working together and on the same side? Birds of a feather–remember?

Demonic spirits panic when you find out who they are and they panic even worse when you know how to get rid of them. Use wisdom when you share what you know concerning them, especially their origin. I thought my family would all receive the news with gladness. It was, at first, some healings even took place, then in time they fled from the truth and hated me for knowing it.

If you can keep the faith of what you know is right the reward will be well worth it. It is an awesome revelation that has brought healing to me more than once. However it totally throws people out of their religious security blanket. I'm still getting hateful looks and nasty letters from family and it has been over 2 years since I let them know who demons are. Why all the hate? I'm sure if I had announced myself as an ax murderer I'd have gotten better reception and a lot more kindness to boot.

Those who knew it was true didn't last too long. They couldn't take the persecution that comes with the knowledge and so they ran away even after some of them bore witness of the truth in their own lives through direct encounters and healings from demonic expulsion....astounding how selfish we really are as human beings and how all our so called 'truth' revolves around us.

Spirit opposes flesh in this world. They are opposites as day is to night being on separate frequency waves. If a person is unwilling to come into the light/HF they cannot receive or hear what you say because it is on a different wave length. That doesn't mean they don't realize that it is true, they will just refuse to know it to be so and they hate you for lighting up their darkness. It is actually painful for them. "Shoot the light bulb or we might see something!" they scream.

I know I'm speaking hard words to hear and if you are still reading it is proof that you want the truth. No one who is completely self involved could have stomached this much truth and still be reading so congratulations seeker of truth may God enlighten you all the way home to heaven's gates.

Can you electrocute an unclean spirit? Yes. You are tuning them in electronically and you can tune them out or torment them, however, it won't be permanent.

If you don't want to reside with them you have to quit tuning them in. When your spirit moves at their frequency level its just like opening your doors and throwing out the welcome mat. They come in when your frequency matches theirs.

There are a lot of electronic zappers out there on the market nowadays and some people live by them; our medical realm is beginning to use them too. They zap the demonic spirit and alter what it is doing but the cure is very temporal as the zappers cannot change what is letting the demon in. How can they? It is your spirit after all. Zappers may mess with the demon's frequency but is not a cure by any means. You cannot evade the Spiritual Laws of God.

No one needs to fear demons. They can only help you do to you what you are already doing to yourself. If you want to be free then you need to align your spirit with God's. You can't do this if you love what is wrong with you can you? So at the root of your wellness, your true salvation, comes the absolute requirement of seeing the truth; repentance. *Every situation has a perfect cause and a perfect cure.* Saying the salvation prayer and going on your way doesn't cut it. Being afraid of burning forever in hell won't save you either. The demons know that Jesus is Lord, hate the hell they are in, live in fear of eternal torment, and they aren't saved. Being afraid that you are wrong won't save you. Salvation is of the Lord....the Truth. Only the Truth known and moved upon in your heart will save your soul. You have to emit HF. Your heart, mind, and soul must be emitting HF.

As long as you are living for God through understanding Jesus, the cross, and true salvation you are the saved. There is no need to worry about yourself anymore. God will take care of you. He never forsakes those who love Him. It isn't hard for Him to save you. It isn't hard for Him to create a new heaven and a new earth. With God nothing is impossible.

Many will seek to enter but only few will be able to because most people simply cannot believe the Truth that they are nothing. They cannot see past the illusions that they love. The illusion of themselves as something, the illusion that there is another way besides God's, the illusion that they are powerful, good, worthy, and amazing. They cannot die to live.

Salvation will only come if you know the Truth in you. You have to admit your sins and see yourself as you really are, not as your pride would like you to be. You have to be able to say, "I was wrong"....help me....and of myself I can do nothing."

You must be able to step away from your pride or you cannot be saved. Prideful people always hate other prideful people, by the way. Arguing—that is where two idiots met and both lost. Hate is a sign of complete pride and jealousy is the cousin to it. Both are based on belief in extreme love and belief in self and not on the Truth that God is everything.

Sliding desperately down a muddy slope to a cliff, grasping with bloody fingers to the wet clay and sharp rocks; this is the feeling that unclean spirits dwell in. They can feel their separation from the Light, feel themselves cold and dark, and they hate the Light. It hurts them and burns the lies that they love. The farther they get the faster they fade into the night. The Truth shining on them is excruciatingly painful as they struggle to survive without Life, hating and cursing Him; they die forever—never to return. This is not the fate that God wishes for you to experience—choose Life. Know that if He had not set a light at our feet that we would not be able to see. What would happen if God decided not to show us anything anymore? Who would save us then? We must be very respectful and obey what we know is right. It would not be good to be given over to a reprobate mind, a mind that has already lost its way in the world. How would we function then? Where would salvation be found? It wouldn't. We must not tempt the Lord our God nor mock the fate of those who have fallen.

Enoch was not and so God took him. He

transcended this world. Every thought has a frequency. What if your spirit no longer emitted a low one? If you move into the higher frequency and into alignment with God's, would you transcend too? Enoch, 'pleased God'. He was aligned completely with Truth. If you or I were to do that, you could literally change dimensions as he did. Jesus said that he could leave at any given time. His life was His to lay down or pick up.

To live in this world and not of it, this was the prayer of Jesus for us. To transcend this world would certainly be to graduate this school called 'Earth' with honors.

It is not that easy to have every flawed thought pulled from one's mind. To seek absolute truth and obey it and have not one piece of false data in ones heart, mind, or soul shows an amazingly humble soul. Obviously it can happen but we see that it is very very rare and the fact that you are present to read this book that I am writing means that we have a ways to go.

Everyone wants to feel their spirit and a power beyond them. This is the part that pulls at my heart strings. If they would only seek the Father's face all kinds of wondrous things would happen. Speaking in real tongues, miracles, and hearing God inside of you....these would be the norm for the day. They would have peace and joy and be able to live above this world and be free regardless of the trials and tribulations. Everything would serve to build you in

Him. Tribulations bring patience, repentance brings the very kingdom that God dwells in, and forgiveness brings salvation. Healing in His wings....the Spirit would come and make His home in your heart. You would be a child of Zion. Your spirit will never know freedom till it is known by God in this intimate way. So what is standing between you and heaven? What dares to steal away life and immortality from you? Deception, lies, unclean spirits, and this world and its ways. This is what stands between you and the Spirit of Truth....between you and your Father.

Every lie you love means that you are just one step closer to hell. Every time you move on what you know is right, what your heart testifies to you, you've moved one step closer to heaven. Which way are you going?

Ghosts already know they are doomed. You see them in photos sitting at their graves bemoaning their choices in life. Some are tragically caught up in the last horrific act that they were involved in on earth before they found themselves in death. Roaming around along side a lost road or shaking the curtains on an abandoned house, you see them trapped, captive in their own thoughts. These are the futures of the lost. These are the pathways of those who chose to believe in themselves. They served the world and spurned what was right and now they lie beneath it. What a gamble. What a foolish foolish game it is to play; gambling one's soul like a handful of quarters in a slot machine.

Ghosts/unclean spirits are everywhere. You see them as orbs, entering and exiting people. The church tells themselves they are angels, they are not. This is yet another disturbing fact for my soul. I noticed that the more ungodly the situation, the more orbs there seem to be present.

You can buy everything from meters to boxes that ghosts will talk in to. There are many ways of communicating with them. The easiest is in your own spirit of course.

Ghosts/unclean spirits cause most of the accidents you see. People have witnessed everything from hands on the steering wheel to illusions in the roadways. Ghosts are rampant but they are not in control. All living things move by spiritual laws. They must abide by God's set of rules. It is like the law of gravity. It applies to everyone. If you should find a way to work around it, then that way exists for everyone.

My final word of advice on being an exorcist? Be serious in your desire to be an exorcist and God will bless you in it, be carnal and you will set yourself for disaster like the Catholic priests who are known for their very 'short' life span.

Nine

Aspects of Spirit Movement

Chakras, auras, and spiritual issues.....

_____

Now that you understand spiritual energy, high and low frequencies, and salvation I would like to cover the aspects of your spirit in greater detail.

First, I need to talk about words. We are a people of 'wordology'. That is a neat word I just made up to describe the science of being word bound. We think with words, know with words, and think we can only discover and learn by them. I would like you to challenge your own wordology and look for the truth behind some words that are commonly used by people who don't have 'bible' words to use. They only have words from their wordology. Words represent concepts. If two people do not have the same concept concerning a word they will not even begin to understand one-another.

I remember the key to success at math. You have to learn to speak math first. This is true with anything and so stepping outside of our 'word' boxes and looking for the concepts and revelations that created the need for a word is often when and where real understanding lies. Such is the case with the word chakra. Christians normally use the word 'spirit' not chakra. However, they are both talking about the same thing. Please read on as I share my story concerning this word.

I had been reflecting on some things that have happened to me and to my delight I have found some words attached to my experiences. Although they are scary words to most bible speakers because they don't have that particular 'word' in their book of learning and they have no handbook of acceptable words and phrases to go by concerning these experiences I ask for grace to use the ones the world uses to tell my story.

Remember, words only mean what you assign to them. This definition is just a little wisdom to help us step past words themselves and enable us to grasp and comprehend the meanings and understandings of what a word is representing. If one were to think, "what idea is attached to this word?"— this is the better way to look at language. Just as we know that America is quite real and referenced to in the bible under differing names, so it is with these words. Just because we don't have the word 'America' in the bible, it doesn't mean that our nation isn't mentioned within the bible or that it doesn't exist.

The concepts that I would like to talk about are

represented by the words chakras, auras, and all the words associated to them. Please realize that the bible is a spiritual book, not a carnal one. It can only be interpreted by His Spirit in you. Carnal Christians are the only ones who actually believe that the meaning of the book is discovered by its letters. These kind always hit you with every translation they can and they spend hours 'debating' to prove their point and sin in the process, trespassing against the very Word they quote. They don't have inward wisdom but only rote, carnal, dead wisdom like the Pharisees to move from so they naturally fight and quarrel. How can they not? They are carnally minded.

13 Which things also we speak, not in the words which man's wisdom teacheth, but which the Holy Ghost teacheth; comparing spiritual things with spiritual.

If you are carnal, moving from pride, lust, greed, envy, doubt, and such you cannot compare spiritual things, you don't have anything to compare it with. You have no spiritual wisdom in your soul. The natural person, the person moving from the ways of this world, cannot receive the things of God/Truth. They are on a different frequency. They may call themselves a Christian, even have a Degree of Divinity, but it doesn't make them spiritual or Divine Minded. Spirituality is only known in you when you are emitting high frequencies and receiving them and has nothing to do with what is going on exterior to your own being.

14 But the natural man receiveth not the things of the Spirit of God: for they are foolishness unto him: neither can he know *them*, because they are spiritually discerned.

Cor 2:13-14 (KJV)

The experiences I am about to share are real and I am not concerned with what Churchianity or the modern day Pharisees have to say about them. I would rather have the Spirit of God moving in my life than ten thousand thousand dead souls with Bible degrees. I do not want carnal man's honor nor do I seek his company. If you are a truth-seeker, may your soul be blessed and your life be enriched as you partake of the body and blood of our Lord and Savior in the wisdom I am about to share. May your life be drenched in peace and joy and wisdom and may your entire being eek with the Holy Spirit!

My Story: I was not seeking anything as far as experience or phenomenon ....I rarely do, but they seem to come and find me instead and often leave me puzzled and wondering till the answer comes.

I was meditating and I began to notice pressure points on my body. The more repentance I experienced, the more these points began to stand out. I wondered if I was experiencing the emergence of new gifts or something. I know very little of other religions, beliefs, and ways and try to keep it that way to keep the information pure and undiluted that I receive from God. This has proven time and time again to be a wondrous decision and I realize now that God led me to do that.

This time, on the following experiences, they came about with a series of strong breaking of pride through repentance and of having my eyes opened up to much of my own sin that I had been moving from. I realize now that this was the beginning of my journey into the Light/higher frequencies that I am experiencing now.

The first thing I began to notice was tingling of body and hands, which I still enjoy immensely, especially while communing with the Father on my bed or sitting quietly in a chair meditating. Then, I began and noticing what feels like a thumb protruding from the center of my forehead and just between the brow area. This came after pressure on the lower back of my head. This surprised me greatly but as usual it took second place to seeking God's thoughts, ways, and His mind. Mind you, all of this is occurring without any prior knowledge of chi, chakras, 3rd eyes, auras, and such. All that information came via other sources at a later date once the experiences brought to my attention that they have been experienced by others, or at least in part.

Several months turned into a year and it is still as strong as when it first happened, actually it has increased in strength to the point that I now feel the pressure down to the center of my nose on to my face and the eye stretches wide across my forehead.

An exorcist I know, thought it was a demon and commanded it back and I felt my head lift and for awhile I thought it was a demon too but then I discovered that he pushed my own spirit back as I can lift the pressure at will. It is my third eye.

My 16 year old daughter is gifted with seeing spirits. She has seen my third eye and said it looks exactly like some draw them, a really big eye in the middle of my forehead. I now have a dent there too! This is so weird. There between my eyes is a very noticeable dent and the pressure is stronger than ever and grows on a continual basis. So here I was, knowing nothing about how it opened and why it was open or what it was for yet experiencing it.

I still do not have a super clear concept of the complete use of that part of my spirit man and am in anticipation of where this is going to lead me as my spirit grows in Him. God has such wonderful gifts for His children. Then, as of late, I have begun to feel a constant downward pressure on the top of my head that prickles and tingles. When the Holy Spirit's presence is really strong, it feels like a thumb. At first I thought that maybe something was wrong with my head, it was so noticeable. I can feel the sensation which resembles small needles pricking the top center of my head quite often. I went and researched it and to my surprise, I now have the crown chakra opened; whatever that meant. I had honestly never read anything concerning chakras. Again, I dismissed it and continued about my way. Apparently, this has been known by the world for many centuries. I'm just a little slow in catching up! This is irrefutable proof that if a person looks for Truth, and not for self, God will always guide one. It is only the pure in heart that can see Him/Truth. God is non-denominational.

I mostly stick to my bible and a few other writings but have not felt the need to look elsewhere and am very satisfied with how the Holy Spirit teaches and leads me. The world is too noisy for me and I really don't like to read a lot; finding words themselves often bothersome and annoying. I'm sure you've noticed my simple language and word usage. I spent much of my childhood sitting by babbling brooks with my little New Testament basking in one verse for hours at a time. I have always loved His Word—His Mind.

The way I have learned of these things is different than most because of the innocence going in to it and no desire to prove anything to anyone. It kept me from basing what I was seeing or experiencing on preconceived notions or the philosophies of others. I have not, nor do I, seek to establish any certain religion or desire to make certain beliefs seem credible. *I do not endorse anything but sincere seeking of God.* I do not seek 'experiences' —they seem to find me and I can see that when one really finds God, one simply 'experiences' God.

True wisdom is simplistic in nature. It is much like a child witnessing a butterfly for the first time. Parents often ruin the discovery process of a child. Why does everything have to have a name, a definition, and an explanation? Why can we just enjoy it the way it is? Have you noticed that people think if they can name something they've overcome it or have experienced it to is fullest? This is foolishness. See the butterfly for what it is. Let it take your breath away without having to pin it to a wallboard and kill it or give it a Latin name so you can deceive yourself into thinking that you now own it. Wisdom from above is not like that.

My journey began by seeing these really neat colors like rainbows around people and things. Pressure points began appearing on my body and I really didn't need a name for it but apparently an earthly word and definition has been attached to the phenomenon and although I will use the words, the explanations are less than adequate.

I found the world's version and description of the things I was experiencing later on and there were a plethora of people who claimed to know all about it, however, I could tell that most only knew about it second hand having little to no first hand experiences. I knew the real meaning was hid in God because wisdom doesn't belong to the self seeker. It only belongs to the children of Truth. How could people who loved sin experience what I was experiencing? God showed me how!

The world defines the Father incorrectly because they seek to use the information to 'better' their flesh and by flesh I mean 'self' or thoughts and ways that are not of Him that dwell in us. They want better health to continue in sin/wrong thinking and to reap more things for themselves on the earth. Do you think that an all perfect God who is without even one incorrect thought or emotion would encourage you into lust or greed or perversion? How about sexual fulfillment or an ambition outside of His way which is the way to eternal life? Perhaps He wants to lead you into a perfect way to get even with someone? Do you think that His mind is behind the schemes to preserve ones 'self' in the next realm so that one can become a god? If you are thinking His thoughts then they will be in alignment with His, won't they? How can you take apples from a thorn tree? Neither can you pick God's fruit from a devil's seed. This is why the world has some information and they use it in wrong and ineffective ways, missing wisdom entirely.

God is with people who love Him. Don't get me wrong here, God is for the salvation of everyone, but you can only be saved by coming into the Light. Therefore it will not be His desire to destroy you but your own desire to destroy Him that destroys you. There are real scientific reasons why this is so. God is completely just and is Life. He isn't playing favorites or controlling people with evil intent. He is Life itself. If you move away from Him, who is life, where do you go?... you enter death...... see? You did it to yourself.

All who honor themselves and live to get what they want based upon the belief that they are a god themselves having a throne, power, dominion, and honor, goodness, power, and so forth, have not known the Truth but themselves as the truth. They created the religions. They serve ideas not the Mind. Just like the useless idols of old, they are made by man's hand, knowing full well they are powerless. The power that is worshiped in them comes from man himself, a projection of his own hopes, lusts, and greed is then worshiped in fullness even to the sacrificing of his own offspring. Purely selfish people will give all that they have to keep the lies they love.

Life in Christ/Truth is amazing! Suddenly— wrapped in His arms, nothing is a threat to you. For God Himself will fail before you do because you are at one with Him. You are honestly standing upon the Rock. It is this Rock of Spiritual Truth that no man can move. The very essence of Reality itself, all the power in the Universe and that which made it is alive in you—what is there to fear? It is because of our sin that we feel shame and from that shame comes guilt and with that guilt comes fear and separation from God. It is sin that keeps us from functioning as we were meant to.

The church that the bible is talking about, His church, are those spirits in whom He lives and when they get together, they fellowship because they have much in common. He is Truth. Is Truth alive in you? Are you honestly leaving behind sin? If you are not, then you are not His church/spirit. His Spirit is to emanate from ours.

This is what chakras really are. I noticed that the sensations of pressure on my crown chakra increased when I would talk about truth, sing, meditate or do a deliverance. My mind was on the Father. It is when my will aligns with His in pureness of heart that the channel and doorway to heaven is open the most to me.

I am going to present my understanding of auras, spiritual energy, and chakras next and hopefully as I understand more I will be able to present it stronger and in a fuller more precise compilation of data to ponder upon as time goes by.

The word 'chakra' means spinning wheel and that is a good description of Spirit energy felt in one's own body at times, especially during meditation, or a quieting of the soul. It does feel like a wheel turning upward and I thought about the design of our DNA. Perhaps it is a physical manifestation of Spirit energy and design. God has no beginning and no end and is much like a circle Himself. So even though the word 'chakra' is tainted with mysticism I will use it occasionally to describe the seven aspects of your spirit.

Our spirits consist of seven spirits or seven specific functions or aspects all intertwined into one, just like our Fathers. We are created spiritual in His image and here is a description of Him.

5 And out of the throne proceeded lightnings and thunderings and voices: and *there were* seven lamps of fire burning before the throne, which are the seven Spirits of God.

Rev 4:4-5 (KJV)

We are created in His image and therefore man has seven aspects or seven separate spiritual aspects which define him. I believe that these are seven levels of high frequencies.

2 All the ways of a man *are* clean in his own eyes; but the LORD weigheth the spirits.

Prov 16:2 (KJV)

This scripture really stood out to me. It begins in the singular sense 'a man' not mankind and says that in effect that God weighs a man's *spirits* as if there is more than one aspect of spirit that belongs to man, and there is.

Should any one of these seven points of spiritual

energy or aspects of man's spirits become fully blocked by sin, we die. This is the sin unto death. It is that simple. Demons enter these areas as the frequencies match and because demons enter, death does too. Should that energy point become fully corrupt it ceases from Life.

The sins that block unto death I believe may be the seven deadly sins mentioned in Proverbs. These sins will be examined in a minute in more detail.

According to what I know, we function correctly and are in health only when we are at least 'somewhat' in alignment with God. The closer one is, the healthier and the further away one gets, the sicker one becomes. Any time we pull away from Him completely in any of these areas—we find death.

Each aspect of the human spirit has a color that is reflected in the aura's that I see. Each color has significance and tells of the state of one's soul. If one color is predominate, then the person is not in moving in harmony with the All Spirit God. The seven aspects of your spirit is what we call the soul. If the soul is not saved it will show up in the aura. The soul is the combination of your experiences for it is your experiences that bring about the choices and thoughts you repeat over and over like a repeater station. All your wishes and thoughts are emitting frequencies and these frequencies have made you who you are today.

I found it kind of amusing that people think their

sin is hidden. Folks, you are lit up like a light bulb!

12 For the word of God *is* quick, and powerful, and sharper than any twoedged sword, piercing even to the dividing asunder of soul and spirit, and of the joints and marrow, and *is* a discerner of the thoughts and intents of the heart
Heb 4:12 (KJV)

Your wish is your prayer. We all pray without ceasing. What are you constantly praying? What are you constantly longing for? These deep longings are about to be answered. If they are not from the right place in your heart, your answer is going to come back to you in a horrible fashion. You will get the wife you always wanted but she will torment you. You will get that house and be so busy working, you'll never get to live there. Everything will be cursed if it comes from a low frequency thought or emotion. Your wishes have made you who you are today and they determine your future. Are you willing to continue on the same path seeing that this is a law of God that cannot be avoided or evaded?

If your longing, your desire, comes from place in your heart, mind, or soul that does not originate from God's Spirit in you, then you are emitting a negative frequency and the demons will bring you your answer. Do you want an answer that comes from the dead and the reprobate?

We see in the above verse that there is a separate distinction between and involving spirit and soul and it is true. Our spirit is like our Fathers, consists of seven separate frequency ranges or bioelectric frequencies and our soul is the sum of them.

Is this the basic elements of who we are, that man consists of seven spiritual energy points which in turn becomes the substance of his soul the entirety of man's being? Does man really consist of seven major spiritual door ways or over all spiritual frequency ranges which must function in unison with the Father's to exist? If these are not in tune or within the range of the Creator's aura or spiritual energy do we die? Yes, we will, and this is what happened to Adam. Death did come to him at once, upon the moment he chose the lower realm/ low frequencies. The very moment he lowered his frequency to a devils, death entered him.

Do we call demons to us by going into lower frequencies? I use the term 'frequency' loosely here as I believe it is something far more complex than what I understand at this moment and so I will say frequency. Some call it biomagnetic or bioelectric, but I don't see the point as they are just words to describe the 'channels' or highways on which spirit operate or moves.

Let's take a closer look at Proverbs 6:12-19.

12 A naughty person, a wicked man, walketh

with a froward mouth. 13 He winketh with his eyes, he speaketh with his feet, he teacheth with his fingers; 14 Frowardness *is* in his heart, he deviseth mischief continually; he soweth discord.

Proverbs 6:12-19.

What I see are seven things happening here.

1. <u>Walking</u> with a froward mouth
2. <u>Winking</u> with his eyes
3. <u>Speaking</u> with his feet
4. <u>Teaching</u> with his fingers
5. <u>Frowardness</u> in his heart
6. <u>Devising</u> mischief (mind)
7. <u>Sowing</u> discord

15 Therefore shall his calamity come suddenly; suddenly shall he be broken without remedy.

This sounds like sin unto death to me....'broken without remedy.'

There is a sin unto death: I do not say that he shall pray for it. 17 All unrighteousness is sin: and there is a sin not unto death.

1 John 5:16-17 (KJV)

213

So we see that a person can get to the point of moving so hard in the wrong direction that it can absolutely cost you your life, lowering you into the demonic realm, the realm of death. Your aura color and frequency will have changed to the point that you die. Not that we can call an electrician and fix it! Obviously, this information isn't critical to the salvation of mankind. I'm just a very curious person who loves to discover God and know Him. He has so many wondrous ways and God delighted me with the understanding of even the mystery behind the rainbow and why people seek to smear that with mockery and sin. More on that later.

Now lets look at the seven things the Lord hates. Now keep in mind that these verses are speaking back to back of the same sins.

16 These six *things* doth the LORD hate: yea, seven *are* an abomination unto him: 17 A proud look, a lying tongue, and hands that shed innocent blood, 18 An heart that deviseth wicked imaginations, feet that be swift in running to mischief, 19 A false witness *that* speaketh lies, and he that soweth discord among brethren.

Prov 6:12-19 (KJV)

This time the same 7 sins are rearranged listed in the order of the chakras.

214

1. A proud look
2. A lying tongue
3. Hands that shed innocent blood
4. An heart that deviseth wicked imaginations
5. Feet that are swift in running to mischief
6. A false witness that speaks lies
7. Someone that sows discord among the brethren

Now, lets make a quick comparison between Proverbs 6:12-14 and Proverbs 6:15-19 in no specific order to prove that they are the same deadly sins:

1. A Proud <u>look</u> >>>>winking with his <u>eye</u>

2. A Lying <u>tongue</u>>>>>walking with a froward mouth

3. <u>Hands</u> that shed innocent blood>>>>teaching with his <u>finger</u>

4. An <u>heart</u> that deviseth wicked

imaginations:**frowardness in his <u>heart</u>**

5. <u>Feet</u> that be swift in running to mischief:
   speaking with his <u>feet</u>

6. A False Witness that speaketh <u>lies</u>: **devising
   mischief**

7. He that <u>soweth</u> discord among
   brethren>>**sowing discord among brethren**

Here we see that they certainly could be one and
the same sins. What is interesting is that they are
listed in the order that they appear to block the
Chakras (spiritual energy points) in the second
listing and I will show you that in a minute.

**The seven abominations in the orders given in
Proverbs 6:12-19 in overview:**

1. **pride/belief in one's self**
2. **lies or lying**
3. **hands that shed innocent blood or
   unjustifiable actions**
4. **heart is wicked**
5. **eagerness to do evil/feet**
6. **planning mischief/conceiving**
7. **sowing discord**

The number seven always means completion or perfection in the bible and I couldn't help but wonder if I was looking at a picture of a completely and perfectly wicked person after reading the 7 abominations.

We are created in God's image and He consists of seven Spirits or aspects of Spirit into one whole as He said in Revelations. Before we get into the aspects of your spirit and the meaning of the colors in one's aura I would like to look at Revelations and I now understand why no one has been able to make sense out of the letters to the seven churches.

1 The Revelation of Jesus Christ, which God gave unto him, to shew unto his servants things which must shortly come to pass; and he sent and signified *it* by his angel unto his servant John:

2 Who bare record of the word of God, and of the testimony of Jesus Christ, and of all things that he saw.

This message is to God's servants; those who seek Truth. It is not to the world or the religious who seek to know themselves as Truth. These cannot hear its content.

Also, people tend to think of the book of Revelations as representing things that are way out into the future yet two thousand years have passed since it was written. The things in this book are things in progress right now as well as future events. It has been the 'end of times' since Jesus ascended into the heavens, has it not?

The book of Revelations is about our souls and the future of the world; speaking of the "things which must shortly come to pass."

3 Blessed *is* he that readeth, and they that hear the words of this prophecy, and keep those things which are written therein: for the time *is* at hand.

This book is a 'now' book. Its pages were just as relevant and applicable to John when he wrote them down as they are to you and I now. You cannot keep, obey, or hear what you don't understand. You have to understand the instructions or the way before you can perform it. So it is in the 'hearing' of it that allows you to keep it. If you don't hear correctly then you won't hear a thing but words and religion. Such is the future of the well educated mind. Hearing occurs in your inner man so if you don't hear this message just ask God to help you and wait upon Him. He must show you in you for you to be able to hear me.

'The time is at hand' means that now is the time to keep these words. Now (today) is the day of salvation. In the present moment is where God is at in your life. This is where you will always find Him. Every spirit everywhere exists in the present moment. They are not gone. They are 'Now". This is where salvation is—in the moment. All who refuse to know it will die in their past. You must come into the present in consciousness to live. This means facing things and being honest and forthright.

4 John to the seven churches which are in Asia: Grace *be* unto you, and peace, from him which is, and which was, and which is to come; and from the seven Spirits which are before his throne;

Asia means that all these churches exist in one major area. They are all a part of one whole. This message is to each aspect of that whole from the seven high frequency ranges of God Himself.

God's own Spirit has seven aspects. These seven aspects of God are 'before' His throne. The 'throne' means that this is the very seat of who He is, where He comes from mentally, emotionally, and morally. It is where he sits, how he sees, and does things. He is based on, from, and upon this place. The Seven Spirits are the essence of who and what He is.

5 And from Jesus Christ, *who is* the faithful witness, *and* the first begotten of the dead, and the prince of the kings of the earth. Unto him that loved us, and washed us from our sins in his own blood,

Speaking of the man Jesus. Who gave His life for us. He was faithful witness of God's character and the ways of God. He only spoke, moved, thought, and emitted high frequencies which makes Him faithful to God. All of His ways/frequencies were correct. He was the first person raised from the dead that God received up into heaven that was perfect in spirit. He now has authority over the spirits of the earth. He cleansed our frequencies by his own blood/vibrations. All who lay down their life for the Truth and pick up His are covered from the wrong thinking that they have. God will not allow their low frequencies to keep them from heaven. As long as they 'carry' their cross, putting Truth first place in their hearts no matter the earthly cost, they will also inherit eternal life. They must lay down their lives to live.

6 And hath made us kings and priests unto God and his Father; to him *be* glory and dominion for ever and ever. Amen.

We will then join Jesus, the Spirit of Truth, one day as we have laid down the desire to create 'another gospel'/another truth/another vibration. As long as we honestly do all that we know to be right in our hearts, God will redeem us from the earth. If not you will join those in death to await the second judgment.

7 Behold, he cometh with clouds; and every eye shall see him, and they *also* which pierced him: and all kindreds of the earth shall wail because of

him. Even so, Amen.

This is most glorious! Know that if you suffer now for what is right that it will one day be 'well' worth it. All the spirits left in the earth, that loved lies, will wail. Why? Because they believed their own lies that they were gods and that they were going to rule the earth. Their mourning comes as the Truth lights up their beloved night.

8 I am Alpha and Omega, the beginning and the ending, saith the Lord, which is, and which was, and which is to come, the Almighty.

Rev 1:1-8 (KJV)

Remember, there is nothing outside of Truth. Truth is all inclusive and can not be added to or diminished from. All who are brethren of Jesus will rule with Him as He rules. And with the rod of Iron, this unmovable, unshakeable Truth will rule all things both great and small. Every knee will bow and admit the Truth as they will all see Him as He is. Every thing that makes a lie will bow the knee to the Truth because Truth will expose it. Hence we will be Kings (people who rule over evil/lies and subdue it with Truth) and Priest (people who understand hearts, plead and intercede for others, thereby helping them come to Truth). This happens in this life, by the way. If you are His, you are becoming and behaving as a King or Priest even as we speak.

9 I John, who also am your brother, and companion in tribulation, and in the kingdom and patience of Jesus Christ, was in the isle that is called Patmos, for the word of God, and for the testimony of Jesus Christ.

This verse just makes my heart sing! "Companion in tribulation"....all who suffer in the flesh, who have abandoned low frequencies, have ceased from sin. All who have denied the demands of self fulfillment and turned a deaf ear to the world and their own selves will know Him/High frequencies in themselves. "In the kingdom and patience of Jesus Christ".....a heart that knows an answer is coming is a heart that can wait. A heart that waits for the Lord/Truth to fix and deal with this world, waiting patiently, looking, hopeful, and with the Truth on its heart and in its mouth, to these the victory will come. They will be found living for the Word and testifying to the Truth as the Truth testifies of them.

10 I was in the Spirit on the Lord's day, and heard behind me a great voice, as of a trumpet, 11 Saying, I am Alpha and Omega, the first and the last: and, What thou seest, write in a book, and send *it* unto the seven churches which are in Asia; unto Ephesus, and unto Smyrna, and unto Pergamos, and unto Thyatira, and unto Sardis, and unto Philadelphia, and unto Laodicea.

Rev 1:9-11 (KJV)

Again, notice that the churches are all in 'Asia'. They are all in 'one' region. This region is your spirit man. You have seven energy points. Those who astral project have seen their spirits attached to one of these seven points.

Here are the seven aspects of your spirit man. Each of these are ministered to by God Himself, His Life Force/Spirit/Frequency. To stay alive you must stay in the high frequency range. He is speaking to the spirits of His children, the children of Truth. Each of the following admonitions applies across the board to every person who has given His life to seek the HF's and has to do with the specific strengths and weaknesses of each energy point. This conversation is pointless with those who aren't saved because they are emitting an overall low frequency. They only have corrupt thoughts and emotions to move from.

God is advising every born again(to high frequency) person to 'keep' the words of His testimony. That means that you are to keep the revelations that he shows you in your spirit man as His own Spirit reveals it. The Churches are your chakras. Before you gasp in horror, let me prove it to you. Be patient with me and read this before you proclaim, "heretic!".

The Seven Churches/Chakras and the definition of their names:

1. **Ephesus > First desirable**
2. **Smyrna > Bitter affliction**
3. **Pergamos > Earthly heights**
4. **Thyatira > Sacrifice of Labor/ Continual Sacrifice**
5. **Sardis > Prince of Joy**
6. **Philadelphia > Love of a brother**
7. **Laodicea > people's opinions/people judged**

The advice given in Revelations is on how to stand in Him in these last days. Even the people who have died will see Him. Every eye will behold Him.

Seven Golden Candlesticks:

12 And I turned to see the voice that spake with me. And being turned, I saw seven golden candlesticks;

John is now beholding the seven aspects of the human spirit. These are your spiritual energy points that are lit and are within His temple just like the

224

ones in the temple spoken of here:

37 And thou shalt make the seven lamps thereof: and they shall light the lamps thereof, that they may give light over against it.

Ex 25:37 (KJV)

This lamp was to light up the temple, just as your spirit lights up your body which is the temple of the Lord. There is much to say here, but I'm going to continue in Revelations for now, bear with me.

These seven candlesticks represent the seven aspects of your spirit man. Pure gold represents purity.

13 And in the midst of the seven candlesticks *one* like unto the Son of man, clothed with a garment down to the foot, and girt about the paps with a golden girdle.

Rev. 1:13

In the midst or very center of your aura is His Divine presence/energy to guide your spirit and correct your energy to His own. This is the Holy Spirit within you who was sent to guide your spirit home. This entity that is in the likeness of the Son of man is God with you. That still quiet voice that says, "here is the way, walk ye in it." The Holy Spirit, the Spirit of Christ is the Spirit of Truth which comes to dwell in all who have given their lives to Him and He dominates or leads those who are His.

Notice again where this entity is at. It is in the 'midst' or middle of the seven candlesticks (which is your spirit). Here is your spiritual 'wheel'. God is the center of your spirit. What you feel spinning is His energy/frequencies rising in your own spirit. Here is how that works.

26 the Spirit also helpeth our infirmities: for we know not what we should pray for as we ought: but the Spirit itself maketh intercession for us with groanings which cannot be uttered.

These groanings which cannot be spoken are His vibrations. When you pray in tongues this energy is being emitted from the center of your own spirit.

27 And he that searcheth the hearts knoweth what *is* the mind of the Spirit, because he maketh intercession for the saints according to *the will of* God.

God is focusing on renewing your mind/spirit. His own Spirit is in yours and is constantly searching your energy points and doing all it can to bring you into alignment. This plan works and will save you if you make an effort to keep the Truth the Lord of your life because it will give the HF predominance over the lower frequencies.

28 And we know that all things work together for

good to them that love God, to them who are the called according to *his* purpose.

Romans 8:26-28 (KJV)

Because you are His, even if you are attempting to follow His thoughts and ways and make mistakes every catastrophe will end up being a life giving lesson. If you always keep trying to love and obey Him. All lower frequencies will come back as an eye opener till you stop emitting that particular frequency. Life will be lessons but not disasters.

The doorway to true spirituality lies just beyond your lusts, the flesh, and this world. All that you need to do to live in peace with the Creator is to submit to what He is saying inside of you right now instead of what the world is saying inside you right now. Every person has this 'Center' in them, whether they tune into Him or not is another thing.

There aren't any people without help....for He is within mankind, talking to him every second of every day. Creation testifies of His character as well. Man will have no excuse for missing salvation. The poor have the gospel preached to them because the truth will set them free from need as you will walk in God's providing hand. All you need is God's Mind in you to move upon and how can you fail? Who can destroy you then?

I believe that the description of the Divine Aura may be relevant to the reconstruction of our own aura. Perhaps someday I will receive a deeper revelation on this, but for now I will put what it appears to be but feel as if I must be honest and say that the Divine Aura may not be interpreted accurately. If I am correct (that this is indeed the aura of God Himself) then each of these characteristics of the Son of man if known in its fullness within us would correct our chakras/spirits and we would eventually be like Enoch—not of this world and gone. Let's take a look at the Divine Aura.

13 And in the midst of the seven candlesticks *one* like unto the Son of man, clothed with a garment down to the foot, and girt about the paps with a golden girdle.

14 His head and *his* hairs *were* white like wool, as white as snow; and his eyes *were* as a flame of fire;

15 And his feet like unto fine brass, as if they burned in a furnace; and his voice as the sound of many waters.

16 And he had in his right hand seven stars: and out of his mouth went a sharp twoedged sword: and his countenance *was* as the sun shineth in his strength.   Rev. 1:14-16

Here is an overview of the Holy Spirit's presence within our own spirit.

- **Clothed with a garment down to his feet and girt about the paps with a golden girdle**

- **His head and his hairs were white like wool as white as snow;**

- **His eyes were a flame of fire;**

- **His feet like unto fine brass, as if burned in a furnace;**

- **His voice as the sound of many waters;**

- **In His right hand He holds seven stars;**

- **Out of His mouth comes a sharp two-edged sword;**

And all these shine strongly. Again, I believe that these aspects that belong to the Son of man are in each born again child of Truth waiting to be made manifest. If known in fullness through revelation, the correction to your spirit man would in fact bring your frequency and the vibration of your own spirit into alignment with God's. If you were vibrating properly, you would look similar to Him because you would know Him as He really is.

Perhaps this is the place to interject that it appears that the armor of God is also based upon correcting your chakras and seems to coincides with the presence of Jesus seen here in Revelations. These are the ways to keep your chakras healthy but lets get back to Revelations and tie this in in the overview of each chakra.

The Son of man, God's perfect presence, the Word, is standing in the midst of your own spirit energy, the seven candlesticks. He's holding the angels/seven stars and shinning in great strength. This means that He is ministering to your Chakras with great strength. When you are aligned with Him you also will be able to minister to others in great strength as His Energy will flow through you to them. Demonic presence will deplete this energy from your spirit which is why some people drain you when you are around them. They have high demonic activity and their aura literally drains yours. Jesus would often go off and re-energize through prayer/meditation. You need to do the same.

17 And when I saw him, I fell at his feet as dead. And he laid his right hand upon me, saying unto me, Fear not; I am the first and the last: 18 I *am* he that liveth, and was dead; and, behold, I am alive for evermore, Amen; and have the keys of hell and of death.

The Spirit of God is Life itself. He laid His right

hand upon John and ministered to John's seven chakras giving him the strength he needed to stand.

Jesus was and is God with us. He had a perfect chakra/spirit because it was God's all the way and was not tarnished with anything corrupt in it.

The 'church' of God is the chakras that are 'His'. It is where He dwells at and resides and is worshiped. Whether you are one person or many, the church, the place where God meets with you, is in your spirit man. The seven aspects of your spirit can be felt easily and I'm going to show you how to do that in a minute but for now lets look at this scripture.

17 And Jesus answered and said unto him, Blessed art thou, Simon Barjona: for flesh and blood hath not revealed *it* unto thee, but my Father which is in heaven.

Heaven is within you. The 'Father', the Spirit of Truth, within Simon/Peter revealed this revelation to Peter, did He not? Because Simon saw the Truth look what Jesus tells him.

18 And I say also unto thee, That thou art Peter, and upon this rock I will build my church; and the gates of hell shall not prevail against it.

Your spirit can only align with God's 'if' you hear the truth in your heart. Your church, your chakra, can only become impervious to hell if it receives and acts on revelations from the Father within you. You cannot receive salvation from outward acts accomplished in your flesh such as attending a church or rote memorization of scripture in order to be saved.

"Repent, the kingdom of heaven is at hand", remember this? You can only join Truth if you have seen it. You cannot mimic it for self gain and fear of losing yourself to death and have it.

The gates of hell, means the way to hell. It will not prevail against the Truth. The Truth will always destroy the lie. Satan has no defense against the Truth in someone's heart. Truth that has been well received will not be moved by a lie.

19 And I will give unto thee the keys of the kingdom of heaven: and whatsoever thou shalt bind on earth shall be bound in heaven: and whatsoever thou shalt loose on earth shall be loosed in heaven.

Matt 16:17-19 (KJV)

Here we see the same declaration spoken in Revelations. All who move from Truth, move from God's very Spirit. Satan cannot stand against those who really are reborn through divine revelation. This is a continual process, not a one time affair.

Earth is the womb. You are either developing into a child of Truth while here or a child of lies. To be birthed into heaven you must be fed from heaven's umbilical cord/HF and then one day you will be birthed fully as you finally see the Truth as He is(the return of Jesus). Should you stop the birthing process completely you will abort the womb, enter death/LF fully, and die. You will suddenly discover yourself in the realm of the dead, blind, and deaf to Truth and if you continue you will head on down in frequency to eternal damnation. The moment you stop the birthing process of continual repentance this is the moment that you begin to really die. God will either rescue you and take you home before it is too late for your spirit or you will be left alone to enter death and fully know yourself as the lie you loved and wouldn't turn from. Those who sin unto death are those who knowingly and loving keep and obey what is wrong for the pleasure of the lie over the love of Truth. These are deep sins blatantly held and adored in the face of God. Unless you repent, there is no where else to go with you but down. You have died in the womb.

Spiritual revelation is the 'Rock' on which the chakras/church stands. This church/chakra/spirit cannot easily be moved by lies/LF as it has received HF of Him in the inward man and whatever it does here by His Spirit is also done in the spiritual realm by God, like a ripple effect. Which is why what you bind on earth becomes bound in heaven and what you loose here is loosed there. This means that what you see and know by Him in you effects this realm just as it does the higher realm. Until you enter the birth canal of God, you cannot begin to know or experience heaven in you.

When God moves a spirit to speak something, the angels uphold it here on this earth as well as in the heavenlies because it is 'God' speaking, not us. We emit His vibrations and they return to us.

19 Write the things which thou hast seen, and the things which are, and the things which shall be hereafter;

The golden candlesticks and the seven stars and churches are things which 'are'. This scripture is speaking in present tense.

20 The mystery of the seven stars which thou sawest in my right hand, and the seven golden candlesticks. The seven stars are the angels of the seven churches: and the seven candlesticks which thou sawest are the seven churches.

Rev 1:12-20 (KJV)

Angels are God's power moving. The candlesticks are your Chakras or spiritual energy points. Each of us have seven angels or aspects that angels work with us on.

We are in the right hand of God because we are the saved. The candlesticks, His lights in the world, are the ones who saw Truth, repented, and cried out for help and mercy and remain in a state of continual growth and repentance. These have received or acknowledged God's Spirit within them and they are following the Good Shepherd into more Truth daily. The unsaved have not acknowledged God's presence in them and are blaspheming him. If they don't turn, they will have committed the unpardonable sin. All who refuse to hear the way things really are, will die.

This message applies to Paul, Peter, and all those who have gone before us as much as it does to us right now. What condition is your spirit in? No one's spirit/chakra has died or gone out. All are anxiously awaiting the 'return' of Christ/Complete Truth. Every spirit everywhere has an aura/energy as we speak and must maintain the Truth in themselves by not following that which is against the Truth. They must stay in a state of continual pursuit of Truth. If you do not heed the warning and your aura is not shining correctly, you are in trouble. You cannot hide it can you? It tells of everything you are and do. It isn't hard for God to keep a data base of all you do. You emit energy and frequencies for every thought and emotion, plus you are glowing. When shining correctly, we are truly lights to the world.

I'm going to go ahead and use the terminology that the world uses for your Chakra points but name them under the real names that God used in Revelations. Then we are going to look at how they work and what blocks them, how the armor applies, and the aspects of correcting one's energy points. Then I'm going to conclude with a meditation exercise to help you sit in God's presence so He can fix yours! Isn't that cool!? And finally I'm going to show you the real 'Law of Attraction' and how to draw *anything* 'Positive' into your life. I want you to see that it is you that determines the outcome of your own life. God made it that way for His own enjoyment. Okay....lets get started!

Below are the seven energy points according to definitions and corresponding aura colors are named below as discovered over the centuries by seekers of Light. First, the name used in the bible by God. Next, the name given by spiritualist. Last, we have the corresponding colors of the aura's.

1. **Ephesus: Mooladhara-red-pink**

2. **Smyrna: Swadishthan-orange**

3. **Pergamos: Manipura-yellow**

4. **Thyatira: Anahata-green/pink**

5. **Sardis: Vishudda-light or pale blue or turquoise**

6. **Philadelphia: Ajna-white/indigo blue, deep blue**

7. **Laodicea: Sahasrara-Violet**

The darker the aura colors the more the auras are tuned to darker frequencies. The lighter the colors, the purer the heart. A really spiritual person will have little color in their aura. It seems to go to greenish yellow, blueish white, to whitish yellow to pure white like the 'hair' on Jesus' head.

Angels are also pure white. Dark red shows up when a person is 'really' worldy. Dark blue going to black is dying. Dark spots in an aura indicate heavy demonic activity and major damage to your spirit. Where the dark spots are at in the aura the person is really really sick in the same place on their body. The demon of death is very noticeable and really big in an aura and often stands outside an aura.

Again, chakras get sick because your life energy force is being shut down by low frequencies you are entertaining. Your mind/emotions emit frequencies, these return to you, which I will cover in greater detail in the 'Law of Attraction' to make sure you haven't missed this aspect of the book. If a body begins to get sick it is because you are pulling death into you through low frequencies. This may be thoughts such as, "I hate myself" or any kind of unforgivable, angry, resentful, greedy, or lustful type of thought and/or any thought outside of God's.

The spirit becomes out of alignment with Life. In order to be well it must come back into alignment with God. Then the body will reflect the spirit. Several things may occur here to heal a body and assist the spirit to a state of health. Repentance, which will bring the sick chakra back into a state of receiving of Life, expelling the demon(s) and then ministering to the person's spirit from the Holy Spirit by touching the person and giving their spirit help from your own aura (virtue), or angelic intervention as seen in highway accidents by first responders where angels lay hands directly on the sick.

In my observation and experience, the strongest and longest lasting is repentance. The reason why is that it will continue to feed the spirit strengthening it daily your spirit grows towards the Light.

The exorcism process is really strong and more immediate for those who are desperately sick. However, the process needs to be done in such a way so as not to scar the emotions as this will cause one to fall into more sin, emitting more low frequencies than before. Therefore, a more tender approach here should be considered and applied due to the dramatic negative effect that can occur. After an exorcism, if a person does not cease moving upon the LF that brought the sickness in, more demons will come to reinforce the wrong thinking making it seven times harder to find the Truth as you chakra lowers. Because the renewing of the mind is hardly an instant process, Jesus told us to 'preach the gospel' and cast out the demons thereby healing the sick. These cannot be separated in the process of creating a well person.

It is possible to restore the spirit energy of a dead body as well and if your energy is correct you can touch those who are sick or dead and restore them again. This proves the Mind over Matter law does indeed exist. God's Spirit moving in you is able to restore the chakra's and vibrations of others. If the Lord is willing for the person to return from the dead, the body can also be restore. It is only a vibration. You must move in accordance to Him at all times. It really is nothing for Him to restore vibrations but He will do so in accordance to His own Spiritual Laws. He is also sovereign, meaning that He has stayed His hand many times when a person humbles themselves in His sight. He only wants what is truly good for you and moves accordingly but cannot deny the Truth.

Casting out demons, healing the sick, raising the dead, preaching the gospel are not separate 'missions' of God, but rather one action occurring on varying levels. God's Spirit is correcting chakras through vessels who bear His in strength. This is why partial healing often take place and why sick people can have miracles come forth from them yet they themselves not be whole. If even one aspect of your spirit lines up, then your aura can help move another's into alignment. This is what we call 'virtue'. Jesus could heal all the sick because He was perfect.

In the area that one's spirit is well, one can assist a healing in another and the the more Truth, God's Spirit, that is in one, the stronger the miracles will be. One revelation moved upon can move a mountain in your life and another persons when revealed to him through you. The gift of healing is an ability to change and heal the auras of another person. Strong green will be in the aura of a person with this gift. A green thumb is also a sign that you have some healing gift present. The plants respond to your touch and vibrations.

It is important to understand that God does not expect you to become perfectly aligned to begin and do His work. He expects you to move upon what ever He gives you and to grow in Him. He is very patient and a good Father. Your mind must become at one with His as will join Him completely one day or you will be without Him. This will not happen over night, but the quicker you move upon His wisdom in you, the clearer you can hear Him, and the stronger your walk will be. If you have the Truth firmly in your heart, who can shake you? No one will be able to remove you from Truth's hand.

God can also 'gift' His presence when He sees fit to do so. He often deems it necessary and gives 'gifts' to some people, even some who are not saved; by that I mean those who do not serve the Truth. Why? He is in the business of reaching souls/chakras. Oftentimes a person will take their gifts and help others into what is right even when they don't know about Jesus. Many in the world do good things from their hearts and they do not know about the son of God. Do you honestly think that these people will spend eternity in hell? You know they won't. God is able to redeem from the realm of death. He has done it before and will do it again.

29 For the gifts and calling of God *are* without repentance
                                           Romans 11:29 (KJV)

God wants you to have life/His frequency and to have it in abundance. He makes things fair for everyone all the time. Sometimes you get rewarded on earth and sometimes in the next realm. He imparts healing and angels according to His wondrous love and mercy. He shines on the just and the unjust. God is gracious and full of mercy and has mercy according to His own pure heart and is not to be questioned in what He does as He is Justice itself. Many ministries have been birthed forth with miracles by the power, love, and compassion for His creation and have little to do with the ministers 'behind' the scenes. Keeping that in mind, I would like to point out that this book is focusing on individual healing and wellness and unity with God through His indwelling presence and not on the subject of healing ministries which are largely angelic presences sent by God's mercy to restore the sick.

Have you noticed that people with a strong negative/low frequency can zap your strength? Some ministries call them 'spiritual vampires' and they are. They seek out really well people to darken. They get their energy to live off of yours. They don't seek repentance, don't want repentance, just your energy to replace theirs. Cruel people get their joy from your pain. They love to draw you into sin. It makes them feel okay about their own sin and allows them to focus on you instead of them.

You know immediately of someone in your own life that absolutely drains you, don't you? What they are really doing is just what it feels like, 'draining your energy'. Right now I know of two ways that you can put a stop to that. One is to avoid the person in daily life if they are really, really, negative and aren't interested in changing and the other is to immediately go pray and meditate to re-energize. If you get too weak, you may sin accidentally by getting angry or impatient because you are tired and then you will get sick. Consider yourself at all times when you help people so that you don't fall with the person who has fallen. Paul knew this and told us to not lay hands on all people and to avoid those who love sin.

22 Lay hands suddenly on no man, neither be partaker of other men's sins: keep thyself pure
1 Tim 5:22 (KJV)

If you move from a low frequency thought you aren't pure anymore. Devils send the LF carriers to you to get you to stumble and sin. Be wary and step away from anyone who loves to sin. Hold your tongue when you are around them and don't extend your soul to them unless the Father shows you that

242

it is wise to do so.

1 Brethren, if a man be overtaken in a fault, ye which are spiritual, restore such an one in the spirit of meekness; considering thyself, lest thou also be tempted

Gal 6:1 (KJV)

Also, I have learned that ministering will drain you. I believe that you are sending out and healing others with your own energy and I have noticed that the more negative people are that you speak or minister to, the more you become drained after ministering. Make time for yourself after preaching or ministering and don't visit for long periods after ministering. Seek to please the Lord in all things, but never harm His Church in you and honor His presence. Let Him lead you in all that you do. Often, you need to separate from people when you feel drained and rest so you can continue in His work and not fall into temptation or tempting someone else. Remember, you are the Church and you fellowship with others. If those whom you fellowship with are lower in frequency you will feel a pull on your spirit or a draining. It will feel much like an emotional drain.

Negative energy has a force behind it which is more of a pull than an pressure. It depletes you and makes you sick and weak. The bible calls it the

spiritual wickedness in high places and that is
exactly what it is. Low frequencies in your 'high
places'.

**12 For we wrestle not against flesh and blood,
but against principalities, against powers, against
the rulers of the darkness of this world, against
spiritual wickedness in high *places*.**

Eph 6:12 (KJV)

What is destroying you is on the inside of you.
Your enemy is within and you feel it. Every power
that draws you from God's energy will kill your
spirit as God's Spirit is the source of all Life giving
energy. Repentance is the key to entering the
kingdom of heaven. It is 'thought and emotion'
realignment. If you want to be a well person you
must seek the Truth, you must seek to know God's
will, emotions, thoughts, and ways. Remember the
spiritual law of seek and find. You will not be
denied the Truth if you seek it. When repentance,
which is turning from an erroneous thought through
revelations occurs in you you stop tuning and
pulling the demons into you. It's that simple.

The rainbow is in the exact order and color of
our auras. I know this is no accident and I have seen
auras in full color and they look exactly like the
rainbow. God's promise to man was given to his
entire being, to his chakra! Man is not flesh, he is

spirit living in a low vibrational body. This will change when he is resurrected to live with Christ/Truth in fullness. God's rainbow is a promise to man's entire spirits/chakras that He would never flood the earth again. Isn't that beautiful?!

The rainbow in the sky is like His signature....a signature of Himself for your spirit man to see. When you look at a rainbow, know that that is exactly what auras look like. Satan tries to blaspheme God anyway that he can and the modern interpretation of rainbows as lesbians and gays is Satan's way of insulting God making rainbows/God's signature a thing to be ashamed of. Satan made it the signature of corruption but to those who know God, the rainbow is still His and represents God's loving heart to mankind, not man kinds perversion and twisted use of one another. I am fully confident that God will destroy even the remembrance of Satan's definition of the rainbow and the word 'gay'. The rainbow belongs to God.

Those who have been given over to inordinate affections—have heart; God can restore anything. What is happening to you comes from things you can't see. Dominate spirits of the opposing sex are often to blame for the strong imbalance but so is the over dominate parent as you seek to overcome their identity in you. Know that you can be whole and well and free. In Christ, there is neither male or female. So if you feel confused as to what a man or woman should be like then just forget both and be

245

neither. Live from truth and it won't matter because Truth is non-gender specific and is not corrupted by the flesh, nor is it defined by this world. Stop trying to please everyone and be either male or female. Love is not sex. Sex is lust. Stop lusting after people and turn your heart to the Truth and you will be free. Do you realize that you are designed to live above this world? You can do it when you invite the Truth into your heart!

What you need isn't in someone else, male or female. You aren't half of a person needing to be fulfilled in another. This is a lie from devils who want you to search for the your needs outside of you as they are hoping to answer your LF. You 'never' needed anyone but the Father in the first place and to find your 'need' in another is to burden that soul with your problems. Any relationship based on using will be miserable. You were designed to find happiness only in obeying the Truth in your heart. All searching for it elsewhere will end in anger and misery.

Distance yourself from this world. Pull away from the 'populace' and seek the Truth with all your heart. Between wicked churches, parents, culture, people, and animals, it is no wonder we cannot find God who is Truth. Stop defining yourself through and by your flesh. Your possessions say nothing of who you really are. Don't ask a stranger to solve your problems...he/she only cares because it makes them feel good. Psychiatry is the biggest con artist job in progress today. Don't waste your money on people who help you only so they can help themselves. This is not God's heart moving these people to 'solve' all your problems so they can feel good and make money off of your pain. When you come clean inside and face your demons in the light of Truth, you will be free. You don't need anyone else.

Chakra points can be felt. Did you know that? Your spirit is the real you. When a person dies, it can be weighed. It can be seen. People astral project all the time and 'leave' their bodies and see the cord of life attached as the venture out and beyond their flesh.

All your problems that seem to come from that body do not. Your body's condition is the product of your spirit's condition and the battle on this earth is only present because you think you are your body and then you foolishly lived as if it were the real you. You then allowed it to dictate your life. You think you must keep yourself well, whole, happy, healthy, and because all things outward appear to affect your body, you assume that all your answers are on the outside of you. They are not.

Everything begins and ends in Spirit. The flesh came about from spirit questioning the Truth. So it is today. All problems arise from questioning what is true or from not having Truth in the first place to move upon.

Flesh of itself is basically worm food. Unable to

effect a single thing, returning to dirt. It is designed to pass away, is momentary and in the realm of death. This is why demons can easily come and go in us. We are both in the realm of death.

Let's take a look at the Chakra points and how your spirit man overlays your physical/LF man. In every place that the spirit is drawing dark energy, or pulling away from the Truth, this will be the place that sickness will enter your body. Cancer is a sign that your cells are dying due to the lack of the presence of Life in your inner spirit man. Instead of denying it, realize that all your woes, trials, burdens, and sufferings have a perfect cure and a perfect cause. Have heart. Like my little 5 year old girl says, "all you gotta do is go back to where you took a wrong turn and go down the right path."

This picture on the following page shows your spiritual energy points. Your entire nervous system is like the highway for spirit movement as this is where you oscillate at in your flesh. There are many nerve points and three known brains in your body; the cerebral, stomach, and heart brain. Treatments such as brain entrainment, acupuncture, and even copper bracelets work because they access and slightly change your frequencies and vibrations. However, the best way to a healthy you is to seek to move upon only God's thoughts and ways. God does not endorse the other ways because they do not realign your spirit and are temporary patches like bubblegum in a leaking dam head.

1 . Blessed *are* the undefiled in the way, who walk in the law of the LORD.

2 Blessed *are* they that keep his testimonies, *and that* seek him with the whole heart.

3 They also do no iniquity: they walk in his ways.
Psalms 119:1-3 (KJV)

Chakra Points

Spiritual Energy Gateways

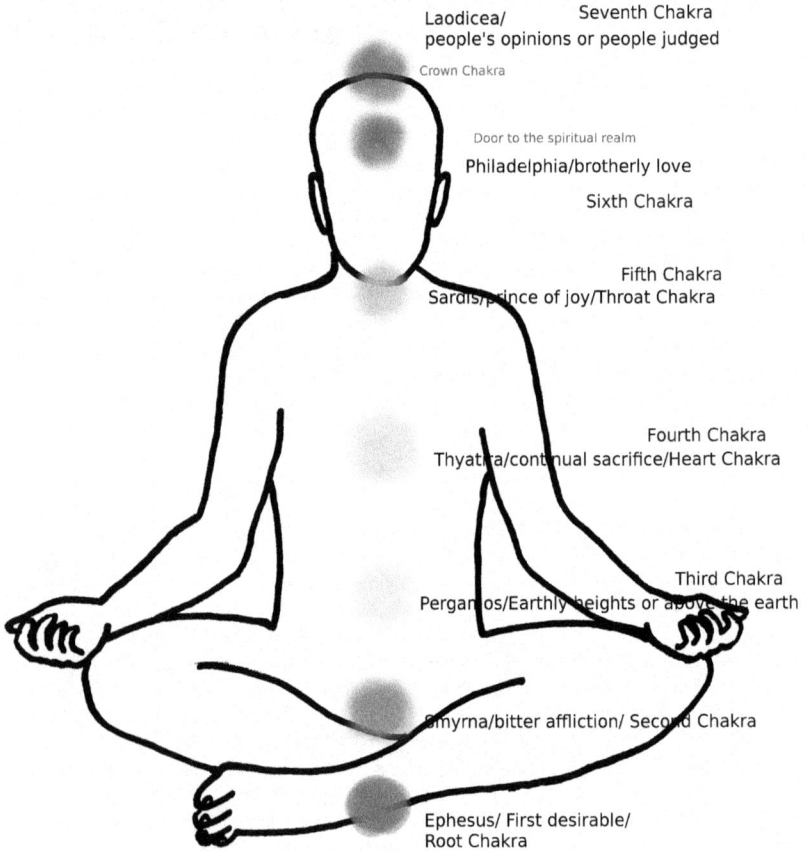

Laodicea/   Seventh Chakra
people's opinions or people judged

Crown Chakra

Door to the spiritual realm
Philadelphia/brotherly love

Sixth Chakra

Fifth Chakra
Sardis/prince of joy/Throat Chakra

Fourth Chakra
Thyatira/continual sacrifice/Heart Chakra

Third Chakra
Pergamos/Earthly heights or above the earth

Smyrna/bitter affliction/ Second Chakra

Ephesus/ First desirable/
Root Chakra

When your energy points become corrupted you begin to die, just like a plant without light. If one of these points becomes totally blocked it won't be long and your body will follow. You killed it, okay? Illness will go into remission from slight repentance. Full repentance would open the door to heal you.

The lower the frequencies you send out the weaker life returns to you and the more cells, organs, and blood in your body start dying. Blocked chakras cannot be cured and cleansed by will; as some are inclined to believe. It isn't you healing you. Your power to get well only comes through Him in you and is a result of His own spiritual law in place in creation. He is the one who sets life and death, right and wrong, before you every day. Then, He gives you the right and ability to make a choice. You do not have the power to fix yourself but only the power to align with either high or low frequencies. Respect His presence as His guidance can end should your heart become too stubborn to see the Truth. We can be given over to a reprobate mind/spirit.

Only that which is correct can fix that which is not. This is the delusion of most people that claim to know all about chakras. You cannot cure yourself with your powers. If you could, then you would be God....and you are not.

I was thinking of Mary of Magdalene. Were her

chakras blocked?

2 And certain women, which had been healed of evil spirits and infirmities, Mary called Magdalene, out of whom went seven devils,

Luke 8:2 (KJV)

Jesus, who is and was perfect in his spirit, was able to restore Mary's spirit. He only did it because He knew she would follow Him and stay well.

Your spirit experiences 'spirit' traffic or movement all the time. If the Holy Spirit is really strong at any given time you may even instantly become unconscious. This is commonly called 'slain in the spirit' by many Christians. This can also occur if a demonic spirit is knocked off of your brain by the Holy Spirit. Temporary unconsciousness can occur.

If a demonic spirit becomes really active, you may fully manifest. When you see someone in a full blown temper tantrum or fit of rage, this usually indicates that the unclean spirit is in charge and in control of the person. Demons also tend to manifest heavily in the presence of the Holy Spirit as they panic and sort of have a melt down. HF's torment them. I can clearly see how technology could fake miracles of God. Perhaps it is already being done and I'm just not privy to it.

There is a word for spirit movement—kundalini.

The word 'kundalini' means vital force or energy. Here is what I discovered concerning the kundalini. It isn't a spirit, as some have taught, it is a word that describes spirit movement. *You hear from the spirit you move from.* The kundalini in you will be the kundalini you move from. If you move from the Holy Spirit you will experience the Holy Spirit answering you and moving in you. If you move from a demon a demon will answer you and move in you. This is the spiritual law of God that we know as reaping and sowing.

The outcome for both is drastically different. One is a channel or doorway to heaven/life, the other a channel/doorway to hell/death.

To tune into hell's channel, just move from something like pride, arrogance, lust, greed, self ambition, or any motive to advantage 'self' and you will have all those spirits who also knew they were amazing gods to show up and help you prove that you are one too. Pride is the foundation of all sin. It is the rudimentary belief that there is an existence outside of All.

To tune into God's channel, move from what you know is right in your heart. A desire to know His mind so you can please Him. To be a better person, so you can be free from sin in your life. You will come from emotions like humility, patience, love kindness, peace, trust, faith, honesty, sincerity, truth, true love, and a deep desire to please the Father's heart.

253

Where you come from will determine where you are going. Past hurts, anger, resentments, all these must be dissolved for you to be healthy because if you move upon these thoughts they will bring demonic spirits into your life. You cannot solve or dissolve them on your own. God's mind must free you from the incorrect thoughts, ways, and emotions that hold you in bondage. This is the beauty of the meditation, but more on that later.

The mantra is the process where the mind is shut down and in this process your spirit is 'sleeping'. Once your mind is shut down, demonic spirits are able to access you freely. The negative kundalini energy is felt in fullness the more you shut down and step aside. One simply cannot come from a selfish wicked place in one's heart and be assisted by the Holy Spirit. An emotion of 'self' improvement to empower your life so you can get everything you lust for will not enact God in your behalf. What will happen is that a demon(s) will enter you through your first chakra, twist and wind its way up through all of your chakras and eventually possess you. The mantra assists them as you open the door wide to them without resistance. They are allowed free and complete access to your spirit and from there, they use your energy points openly. This is one way to become fully demon possessed, by the way. To guard against the spirits of this world we are told by Jesus that we must 'watch and pray'. We are not to go to sleep spiritually and allow other entities to enter and do as they will nor are we to let what is 'outside' of us lead us. To tune into the correct spirit you simply need to be humble enough to be honest about what God shows you, that's all. It takes no special talent, no amazing ability but only a willingness to follow the Truth and a contrite and humble attitude.

Tongues speech is much like the mantra. It causes your frontal lobe to also 'step down', the difference is that God's indwelling presence takes over whereas in a mantra a devil's presence takes over. As you pray in tongues your frequencies are being changed and aligned. Paul said he prayed more than everyone in tongues. Perhaps we should pay heed.

The advice given by many concerning chakras and spirit movement is extremely harmful. Many consider the chakra fully open and working when one is in the state of full demon possession. Most teach that a chakra is not fully open it unless you are involved rigorously in pervert sexual acts and other 'flesh' fulfilling activities. The information concerning mediation and chakras available to the public is by large demonic and the secret to a working chakra will never be discovered by minds that do not know the Truth.

Now that we have discovered the meaning of the chakras, energy, angels, stars, candlesticks, and kundalini, lets go on to the way your spirit functions. We will look at each aspect of your spirit and what must occur to align you with God in you.

Ten

Your Energy Points

Energy points, comparisons, and wellness

1st Chakra>Ephesus>First Desirable

The word Ephesus means 'first desirable'. This is your first chakra or first awakening of your spirit/ church. Your new creature was born and birthed from the very first desire you had to hear and obey the Truth from your heart. You saw your sinful nature, did you not? You saw that Jesus died for you and you were not worthy. In a moment of humble contrition you realized the truth in your heart of who you were and believed what you saw. This conviction, inner knowing, is what you must heed to continue towards heaven's gates. The moment your first chakra began to function somewhat in accordance to the inner Light by repenting was the moment your spirit was born again. It moved from lie loving to truth loving. We are born of Spirit, led by Spirit, and His Spirit dwells in us.

13 Hereby know we that we dwell in him, and he in us, because he hath given us of his Spirit.
1 John 4:13 (KJV)

In obeying the Truth from the heart, you found Him in you. Love, Light, and Peace as you had never known flooded your soul and you knew what it meant to be 'saved'. You obeyed the Truth from your heart. This is the shining moment that caused you to plunge into water and come out a new man (baptism). Your inner moving towards the Truth caused an outer movement as testimony of the inner Light.

By outward manifestation, you denounced the world and its ways by going under the water as to the grave and then in your rising your 'new' man burst forth in shining Light, the chakra was, in that moment, a new creature in Christ Jesus, was regenerated by His Spirit, you are now 'Spirit led', whereas before you were flesh or demonically led.

So here you are, this new baby, born of Truth, in a world that hates you. Pardoned by the blood of Jesus, birthed as a new creature in Him. God's Spirit has awakened your own and you are now a 'light' to the world's chakras. You are that candle that cannot be hid; a testimony of His own Spirit.

Here is what the Spirit of Christ has to say about the first chakra, the dangers it faces and its challenges in the world.

1 Unto the angel of the church of Ephesus write; These things saith he that holdeth the seven stars in his right hand, who walketh in the midst of the seven golden candlesticks;

(Rev. 2:1-7)

He's reminding you of your origin saying that you now come from a place of Truth in you. The Truth is now in your midst.

2 I know thy works, and thy labour, and thy patience, and how thou canst not bear them which are evil: and thou hast tried them which say they are apostles, and are not, and hast found them liars:

A person who has turned away from the lies in his/her own heart finds it really hard to happily entertain people who love lies. You find the lies amongst those who say they are His but who really aren't really egregious. They are nearly unbearable and completely obvious to your heart and soul.

3 And hast borne, and hast patience, and for my name's sake hast laboured, and hast not fainted.

Even with all the persecution from the world and from those who say that they love God, but they hate the Truth, you have stood your ground. It took effort and much endurance to bear the scorn and persecution. You have not quit for Truth's sake and have remain faithful to what you knew was right in at least some measure. You have endured scoffing, cruelty, hardship, and pain and exclusion from the world for refusing to join in their games, philosophies, and sins and also from Churchianity for not playing the part of a Pharisee. You in essence have found yourself a pilgrim in a world gone mad.

You didn't let people guilt trip you, you rose above their criticism, endured their mockery, peer pressure, and you turned the other cheek. You have labored to walk the straight and narrow path even at much personal cost to you. You did not defend yourself, you did not take revenge, you did not seek your own glory, your laboring is not in vain. When you are like that, the chakra is near perfection or functioning perfectly. It is keeping its 'first desire' which was to know the Truth at all cost to self. Here is its weakness.

4 Nevertheless I have *somewhat* against thee, because thou hast left thy first love.

The weakness of this first aspect of your spirit is that you could lose your first love/desire. In other words, you leave behind your desire of Truth. If you meet someone who speaks lovingly of their born again experience but then says they are in a 'dry' period, you can be sure that they left their first love. Forsaking the first commandment is your big danger. This is what shuts down this energy point and will cause your chakra to become out of balance spiritually and fail.

Giving in to what you know is **not** right for fear of the burdens that one must bear is the main reason that people leave the Truth behind. They could not endure the persecution and temptations and fell back into their flesh. The dropped their cross. Giving in to their lusts and the world, they forgot the love of Truth that their heart once knew. They lost their first love.

Stop for a moment and reflect on how strong the pull is to go back to loving deceit. Hate is in every heart around you, everyone's competing, living like there's no tomorrow. Our society is extremely liberal, thinks nothing of killing a baby and licensing every kind of evil under the sun. You, my friend, do not fit in. In your lonely state, you are tempted to fall into relationships that make you weak (if you are not already in one) and after a while of getting hit from the religious and the wicked, you've pretty much had enough of both.

5 Remember therefore from whence thou art fallen, and repent, and do the first works; or else I will come unto thee quickly, and will remove thy candlestick out of his place, except thou repent.

They key word is that He will come 'quickly' to remove your candlestick. God doesn't hang around people who love lies and practice devil ways; lust, hate, greed, arrogance, pride, etc. He knows the proud from afar. Be quick to repent. If you do not have a love or understanding of Truth then your candlestick will be removed. That happens 'now'. Many have had theirs removed and He no longer lights them. They live in darkness and they are growing sicker day by day in their dead religions. These people usually portray strong pride, fear, doubt, greed, and anger while spouting God's name. They are spiritually blind.

A sign that His candlestick is about to be removed is extreme misery in your soul. You will find yourself trying to fulfill your own self through others and outward means and it will usually have strong sexual or dominating overtones as you try and fulfill yourself through others. You will also behave with animal type behavior such as fight or flight as you are not drawing your understanding from the Guiding Light within. A tendency to know yourself through self-realization like putting others up on a pedestal and living unto them and infatuation are signs that your 'first love' is not the Truth but yourself. If you think of yourself all day long, worry, or fret, you are your own god. It is you trying to fix everything and be everything. Although you are feeling the truth of your nothingness in the subconscious mind you refuse to submit, lost your first love and now live from worry and fear.

There are many who say they are Christ's and they are not. They are just 'religiously' in love with themselves in His name. These are already without candlesticks or near removal. In many cases it was never really lit. They never had a foundational love of truth.

6 But this thou hast, that thou hatest the deeds of the Nicolaitans, which I also hate.

God recognizes that it was because you hated evil in the first place in yourself that caused you to hate it in others and this is what brought you to the Truth. This is basic salvation and where all believers start at. If they stay there and continue to build upon that foundation then they will overcome the world in themselves and successfully be faithful unto death of self and receive the crown of Life. However, if they do not carry their cross and die faithfully to this world, but self/flesh comes fully alive again they are not Christians any longer, but Pharisees. Religious folks who use Him for self gain.

Niclolaitans means 'ruler of the people'. Basically, sin rules people and when you hate the deeds of sin which God also hates it means that you love the Truth.

7 He that hath an ear, let him hear what the Spirit saith unto the churches; To him that

**overcometh will I give to eat of the tree of life,
which is in the midst of the paradise of God.**
Rev 2:1-7 (KJV)

Whoever can keep the love of Truth will
overcome this world. One must not let go of what
one knows is right. These, the overcomers, will be
able to partake of Life because they hated the way
of sinners(wrong thinking and emotion) and they
bore the persecution of it in the earth even though
the price was often very high.

Malfunctioning Ephesus: Moments of extreme
fear, panic attacks, and flight or fight instinct really
active....they are mad one minute and arguing and
then running the next, insecure, resentful, extremely
self centered, fear based mentality, and have a self
preservation mind set. Arrogance is why they cannot
see and it is their deep love of self that keeps them
in the dark/low frequencies.

Functioning: Purity, innocence, feeling secure,
much dignity, patient, confident, able to endure, no
desire to use people, willing to not look to others for
what one needs but secure in that God is one's
provider. This is the root chakra, like the foundation
of the others, you build up from here or come from
this place in all that you do. A good solid
understanding of the first commandment would

keep this energy point well because you wouldn't be using anyone or needing any approval and you would serve the Truth. More than likely you will find yourself between the two examples in a place of growth.

If you actually analyze your own behavior you will see that you have worked quite hard in your life to be naughty. You day dreamed about it, spent hours perhaps months grooming your appearance to catch that babe for that one night stand. Look at all the effort that goes into a well laid out crime! Imagine if you put all that energy into finding and doing God's will.

The problem is when your heart is wicked your life will follow suite. Purity of heart is the only way to see Truth. Many who seek to enter the kingdom of heaven do it for self gain and it cannot be done that way. Self has to die and it can only die in the light of Truth. One cannot ambitiously destroy all the wrong thinking in ones self because we are not the source of the Truth, He is. Therefore, to take it upon your shoulders to cure yourself is impossible. Only pride would attempt it. You must be able to humbly come to God and ask, seek, knock, and then wait. God must impart Himself in order for you to be well. This is where bible studies harm people. They get up in their pride(wrong thought) and seek to acquire some more 'God' in them. What they receive will not bless them but destroy their true spirituality because they moved from a negative emotion— pride. You cannot worship and serve yourself and God at the same time. You can, however, serve yourself in His name and pretend to be saved, but it does not make it so. Why do you do what you do? Ask God to help you and to purify your heart. Only He knows what needs to go and what needs to stay. He is the Way.

To keep that chakra healthy you have to love the Truth and not lay it down for anything. I'm not talking about the 'kind' of truth where you are your own truth and make up doctrines and religions. I'm talking about seeing things the way they really are in humility and contrition. You will live in a state of 'continual' repentance. Every day, moment by moment, you will be turning from wrong thoughts to correct ones. This is how you grow in Christ/Truth.

I know I'm somewhat repetitive. I feel it is crucial for you to understand the definition of Truth as so many ministers mean 'the way I see it' instead of 'the way it really is.'

Snapshot

1ˢᵗ Chakra : Ephesus/ First desirable

Color: red to pinkish, people with strong dark red tend to be really worldly and close to death.

Location: base of the spine

Sicknesses: Lymph system, skeleton system (teeth and bones), the prostate gland in men, the sacral plexus, the bladder and elimination system, and the lower extremities (legs - feet, ankles , etc.). Also the nose, since it is the organ of the sense of smell, and associated with survival.

 Deadly sin that can block it: pride/belief in one's self which uproots the first commandment and was man's original sin

Corresponding Armor: feet shod with the preparation of the gospel of peace

Divine Aura: feet like unto fine brass

(Being at peace with the Truth in humble contrition and firmly standing upon what you know is right is the key to keeping this chakra point healthy)

2cd Chakra>Smyrna: Bitter Affliction

8 And unto the angel of the church in Smyrna write; These things saith the first and the last, which was dead, and is alive;

Rev 2:8-11 (KJV)

God promises from His own mouth to those in bitter affliction, suffering in their flesh, to remember that He is the first and the last. The Truth is all that there is therefore He is the beginning and the end of all things. Just as Jesus died to His flesh, rose again, and is alive with the Father, sitting on His right hand. You are to do the same. You can only come to the Father through Christ, the Spirit of Truth, and only those who do as He did in the earth are those who will abide with Him forever.

9 I know thy works, and tribulation, and poverty, (but thou art rich) and *I know* the blasphemy of them which say they are Jews, and are not, but *are* the synagogue of Satan.

Notice that God is 'rehashing' the condition of the church of Ephesus. He is recapping. Some of His people will suffer more than others when it comes to persecution. And again, He remembers how the religious persecute Truth seekers.

10 Fear none of those things which thou shalt suffer: behold, the devil shall cast *some* of you into prison, that ye may be tried; and ye shall have tribulation ten days: be thou faithful unto death, and I will give thee a crown of life.

God is saying, "Don't be afraid of the things you must suffer. Demons will try and punish you for obeying Me, they will do everything they can to keep you from doing that which is right and good. It is this way so that what you understand may be tested, however, your suffering will only be for a short while, like 10 days compared to your life span. Be faithful unto death; be faithful to the truth and die to your flesh and I will give you life."

People tend to misinterpret the meaning of death. There are many living dead amongst us. Death is of spirit, not flesh. Flesh is temporal and your flesh as you know it now will never be restored. Death for some will be permanently known because they loved not Life.

Being faithful unto death doesn't necessarily mean of your flesh as martyrdom but more specifically in your spirit. Who are you 'alive' to? Are you living unto the Truth or lies? Whose mind are you living from? Are you dying to the thoughts and ways that are not of Him....like selfishness, greed, lust, envy, etc.? If you are and are dying daily (suffering bitter affliction), then you are being faithful to the Truth and your flesh/low frequency ways are now dying in you. You have to die to the LF and be reborn to HF. Only those who die can truly live. This is not a one time process but a 'daily' process. Should you ever cease from the repentance process you have lost your salvation.

The problem that comes from this chakra is that of endurance. Can you hold on to your 'first desire?'.

11 He that hath an ear, let him hear what the Spirit saith unto the churches; He that overcometh shall not be hurt of the second death.

He is saying, "For those who are already dead to the world and alive in Me/Christ, there is no second death. For all those who love themselves above Truth, these will really die. For all lies will return to the void/dust from whence they came."

When this spiritual energy point or aspect of your spirit is working properly you will have truly laid your life down for the Truth. This is a surrender of the emotions and of the will—it can only be done through divine revelation.

If you are willing to endure for 'ten days' or a short while and die to your flesh you will receive that crown of life. That crown is your 7th chakra which is your divine connection to heaven itself.

To have it fully opened, you must be fully able to die to your flesh and endure the temptation and persecution of the worlds thoughts in the low frequency range otherwise you can kiss goodbye to living in and by the Holy Spirit.

Malfunctioning: Self gratification, an unwillingness to suffer for what you know is right. Also may show up as self hatred. Blaming yourself when your godhood fails. **You** are the center of your world. You love yourself when you succeed and hate yourself when you feel you've failed.

Functioning: Pleasing the Father, sacrificial, patient, quiet, calm, humble, and willing to suffer and endure. You have tasted the 'bitter affliction' that comes from being at one with Truth in a world that hates Truth. You've endured it.

If you are sick are in the areas mentioned in the 'snapshot' it probably means that you are not doing what you know is right and your mouth is out of control. You aren't willing to suffer for righteousness sake. Instead you 'get even' and tend to move from low frequency thoughts. You don't know bitter affliction.

The bible says that we eat from the fruit of our mouths.

20 A man's belly shall be satisfied with the fruit of his mouth; and with the increase of his lips shall he be filled.

Prov 18:20 (KJV)

19 Wherefore, my beloved brethren, let every man be swift to hear, slow to speak, slow to wrath: 20 For the wrath of man worketh not the righteousness of God.

James 1:19-20 (KJV)

A mouth that doesn't speak the truth that the first chakra has come into an understanding of will shut down this chakra point. Death will come in the areas listed above, especially in the reproductive organs. Life will not be flowing in through this chakra like it should and your flesh will begin to get sick.

This is one reason so many women get in trouble. They are always gossiping and slandering to hurt other people instead of suffering for what is right. They play God and seek to punish according to their own ideals.

The nastier your mouth, the sicker this chakra becomes. Some women are barren. Their mouth is most likely 'way' out of alignment. This aspect of your spirit must come into alignment with God. You must become willing to suffer for what is right and that means that you must stop playing god in other people's lives.

If you will quiet down, be humble, listen to the truth, stop trying to get revenge, punish and reward people, and suffer in your flesh for that which you know is right then you will enter the kingdom of

271

heaven and be well. The suffering is really not that long before the hug of your Father comes to rescue you. If people only knew!

Give up that candy bar temptation to gossip, let go of that moment of revenge. Be willing to suffer for the Truth; for what is right. The person who suffers this way does not sin (move upon wrong thinking.) A revelation of the Real Law of Attraction would help cure this chakra.

1 Forasmuch then as Christ hath suffered for us in the flesh, arm yourselves likewise with the same mind: for he that hath suffered in the flesh hath ceased from sin; 2 That he no longer should live the rest of *his* time in the flesh to the lusts of men, but to the will of God.

1 Peter 4:1-2 (KJV)

Look at the corresponding armor below in the snapshot. Your heart isn't in the right place which is why you can't stop your mouth. To keep it healthy? Watch your mouth! Bring your heart before God everyday and seek the truth of its real status. You can't be taking revenge and speaking evil of others and be enduring persecution at the same time. You are the persecutor! You must suffer 'bitter affliction' which means you can't be the afflicting person.

272

The reason you aren't able to endure is because you aren't secure in Him. You are worried about what other people think. Pride plays a huge role in what you are doing. Understanding that revenge is unnecessary would also really help this chakra.

Snapshot

2cd Chakra : Smyrna/bitter affliction

Color: orange...the darker it is the more worldly you are and the closer to death you are coming

Location: lower abdomen/lower back (below navel)

Sicknesses: reproductive system, sexual organs, lumbar plexus. liver, kidneys, and the lower abdomen

Deadly sin that can block it: lies/lying and a froward mouth

Corresponding Armor: sword of the Spirit

Divine Aura: mouth goes a sharp two-edged sword

(The opposite of lying must occur. One's mouth must speak and move within and upon the Truth; His words, thoughts, emotions, and ways.)

3rd Chakra>Pergamum:

Your third chakra is called Pergamum and it means 'earthly heights'. When this chakra is not functioning in harmony with God you are in 'big' trouble. Demonic spirits usually work from this area.

A person for instance who gets angry can feel the spirit rise from here in your solar plexus. It is the reason for uneasiness, short breathing, and trembling and nausea. This is where most demons sit and where I find them during exorcisms. They use the stomach brain which is the seat of your emotions. Scientist have proved that there are three brains in your body—stomach, heart, and the cerebral. Unclean spirits use your brains and can get you to do things and imprint not only ideas, thoughts, and ways but their own emotions.

Infants are able to have a fully functional body 'before' a cerebral. So I know that the stomach brain is capable of doing much. Demons operate on low frequency and use your brains much like a person does a computer. They can feel and see through you by accessing your brains. For demonic possession to occur the demon must overlay your brain and control your crown chakra.

12 And to the angel of the church in Pergamos write; These things saith he which hath the sharp sword with two edges;   Rev 2:12-17 (KJV)

There is an amazing amount of information in the following scripture.

13 I know thy works, and where thou dwellest, *even* where Satan's seat *is*: and thou holdest fast my name, and hast not denied my faith, even in those days wherein Antipas *was* my faithful martyr, who was slain among you, where Satan dwelleth.

Demons sit in the belly and rise and fall from there. That is why this is 'satan's or the devil's seat'. For those who are resisting devils and have held fast to His name and have not denied Him, they are the 'Antipas'.

Antipas means 'against all'. If you are able to fully resist all demons, or as Paul says 'your flesh' then you are the slain and faithful to the Truth in you and you are a faithful martyr. You have to rise above the frequencies of the earth, hence 'earthly heights'.

14 But I have a few things against thee, because thou hast there them that hold the doctrine of Balaam, who taught Balac to cast a stumblingblock before the children of Israel, to eat things sacrificed unto idols, and to commit fornication.

The weakness of this chakra is taking the teachings of devils or the minds of the religious and following them into sin. You are holding the doctrines of Balaam. Doing so will put a stumblingblock in your way and you will digest, take in and live from things that are abominable to God.

Balaam means Destroyer Of People, or Confuser Of The People referring directly to devils themselves within groups of believers, especially those caught up in Churchianity. In Psalm 55:10 this verb is used to mean confusion, much like the verb *balal,* meaning to confuse or mix up people.
So we see that Balaam comes from a spirit that confuses people to devour them and it is a religious spirit.

Balac/Balak is the son of a Moabite. Moab is the incestuous son of Lot, a righteous man. Moab means 'who is your daddy?'.

This verse then says, **"But I have a few things against you, because you have there, in your belly, them that hold the religious doctrines that originate from devils/satan, who taught those who didn't know Me to cast a stumblingblock before the children who did, to eat things sacrificed unto idols (self idolization), and to commit fornication (loving religious lies over the truth) for self advantage.**

This would include such teachings as the prosperity message, self realization through church titles, degrees, and such. Teaching that it is okay to be wealthy in a starving world, self worship, blab it and grab it (which is nothing more than coveting), fear of hell as basis for salvation (brainwashing), and all such abominable teachings.

15 So hast thou also them that hold the doctrine of the Nicolaitans, which thing I hate.

Again, from before, we learned that the Nicolaitans are those who love and practice sin or wrong thinking. The Truth hates lies. God is saying, "from this place you also have the teachings of the lost which I hate. You have been duped by religious people/spirits into believing things that are not of me."

16 Repent; or else I will come unto thee quickly, and will fight against them with the sword of my mouth.

The truth from His mouth will destroy that which is not true. If you do not align yourself with Him, you will be destroyed.

If you don't turn from the wrong ways, the ways of lies, false doctrines that you invited into your midst because they appealed to your flesh you will perish with the lies. Deceit, selfishness, greed, hate, lust, and a desire to be amazing are the ways of Satan. Any preacher or person who claims they are of God but teach the ways of Satan are going to be destroyed by God one day soon. Do not align yourself with anyone who loves to move on religious wrong thinking for self advantage. If you do such a thing, God's own aura will disown yours. You will die from separating from Him. His Truth will not mix with the teachings of devils or the world.

17 He that hath an ear, let him hear what the Spirit saith unto the churches; To him that overcometh will I give to eat of the hidden manna, and will give him a white stone, and in the stone a new name written, which no man knoweth saving he that receiveth *it*.

If you can hear the Truth, obey the Truth, and overcome the devils who have access to your aura then you will partake of that 'hidden' manna, the spiritual revelations that are able to sustain you. Your relationship with your Father will be a personal experience and you will truly know Him personally.

I have found this to be true! Oh my gosh, I am a living testimony and I don't care if everyone calls me names or hates me. God's true word is hidden from the hypocrite who bears God's holy name for self gain. The eyes that are wicked cannot see and the ears that love lies cannot hear. Go ahead and disown me world cause I love my Father and I don't care!

279

Malfunctioning: Illness as listed in the snapshot. You will feel activity in your solar plexus, trembling, queasy sensations when you do something wrong or when the unclean spirits accessing you feel endangered. Twitching, especially facial. Loss of appetite triggered by depression or anger, clenched teeth which correlates with tightened stomach muscles, acid reflux, diarrhea, etc.

You will feel a rising of hatred, anger, and a blurry minded blood rushing sensation to the head when an unclean spirit rises. Often people do things they really regret when an unclean spirit manifests strongly while in that state. Many have trouble recalling what they said or did after a manifestation. The reason why was that it was not their mind involved. They were 'full' manifest.

Emotions such as greed, lust, envy, jealousy, also come from this area. Blind rage, and a cold dark sensation are the spirits present that are in or near you. Because the solar plexus is a complex network of nerves demons tend to congregate in this area. Acupuncture does actually help control their frequencies but God is not pleased with these things. If you are a Christian He expects you to become well in Him. He 'alone' is your Savior. If you want relief from demons you have to quit congregating with them and renew your mind in Christ. You must begin to repent of all the thoughts and ways that are incorrect—as he reveals them to you.

Functioning: You would be able to clearly hear His voice and obey. You would be moving from intuition, wisdom, and rising above this world. You should feel a stirring and rising sensation of God's emotions from your solar plexus: love, peace, tranquility, serenity, joy, calmness, patience, and gifts of the Holy Spirit. You will have risen above this world. Paul told Timothy to 'stir up the gift that is within you.' This is the place it is stirred up from.

Snapshot

3rd Chakra : Pergamum/Earthly heights or above the frequency of the earthly

Color: yellow; the lighter it is, the more correct your chakra. Dark yellow would be a sincere love of communication with the demons. People who tend to communicate easily with spirits often have much yellow in their auras

Location: solar plexus and associated nerves

Sicknesses: muscles, stomach, digestion, pancreas, liver, gallbladder, metabolism and the nervous system. Pancreatic cancer, nerve disorders, gastric problems, renal, testicular, spleen, etc.

Deadly sin that can block it: hands that shed innocent blood (actions based solely on demonic impulses)

Corresponding Armor: loins girt about with truth

Divine Aura: clothed with a garment down to the foot

(Loins was always referred to in the bible as a place where a child(spirit) was birthed forth from. Instead of birthing the actions of unclean spirits into your life you are to birth Truth and be clothed in Truth.)

4th Chakra>Thyatira

In this chakra you will see a very serious message from Christ. This is the heart chakra and it is with the heart that man believes unto salvation. Listen to the rebuke:

18 And unto the angel of the church in Thyatira write; These things saith the Son of God, who hath his eyes like unto a flame of fire, and his feet *are* like fine brass;

Rev 2:18-29 (KJV)

He is saying to your heart. I see you exactly as you are and I'm not moving from what I see.

19 I know thy works, and charity, and service, and faith, and thy patience, and thy works; and the last *to be* more than the first.

Your works/heart are improving.....However.....

20 Notwithstanding I have a few things against thee, because thou sufferest that woman Jezebel, which calleth herself a prophetess, to teach and to seduce my servants to commit fornication, and to eat things sacrificed unto idols.

Jezebel means 'false teacher'. She turned the king away from God, was a manipulative woman who did more than anyone to promote an evil religion. Thus, in Christian tradition, a comparison to Jezebel suggests that a person is a pagan or an apostate masquerading as a servant of God, who by manipulation and/or seduction misleads the saints of God into sins of idolatry or sexual immorality, sending them to hell. These are the false teachers in the body of Christ who live to promote evil within people in the name of God. False teachings, prophecies, writings, and those who claim they are His servants and are not.

The biggest danger to your heart chakra comes from believing the lies of these people and are those within the church who are sinning and making it appear as though God approves.

The more 'religious' a person is, the more Jezebel lives in that person. Those who want to become Jezebels themselves are the hardest ones to pull away from lies and self worship. They worship people because they want to be worshiped. They are fully in love with themselves in God's name and their religion is all about them.

Fake preachers, evangelists, pastors, prophets, and teachers, are everywhere! If you haven't noticed and cannot pick them out you should ask yourself why that is?

21 And I gave her space to repent of her fornication; and she repented not.

God will give you time to see the truth but if you

284

don't he'll give you over to that reprobate mind that you loved to entertain. Fear is the beginning of true wisdom for in respecting the Truth in your heart you will find God.

22 Behold, I will cast her into a bed, and them that commit adultery with her into great tribulation, except they repent of their deeds.

To take up sides with religious demonic spirits (which is the center of the Jezebel spirit) one must 'sleep' or become intimate with devils. This is adultery because you were once intimate with your Husband, the Truth, and now you take to bed with devils and follow their leading for self gain...all because you had to be important or special. The reason this is such a problem for you is that you followed God to be important. This is the heart of the Jezebel Christian.

You wanted the lie that they teach. You wanted to see that you are good, special, and amazing...just like them. You love to believe that you can be completely arrogant and saved. It is okay to be just like the world as long as you say, "Jesus is Lord." Heck you can do anything! You can be wealthy, healthy, wise, powerful, proud, and everyone will want to be just like you and see how wonderful you really are. All those fights and debates just prove how smart you really are. You demand to be called by your title, Dr., Pastor, Apostle, etc..You have the only true religion in the world. Wow, you are amazing! This is the corrupt Jezebel mind. You cannot become God no matter how you try and you will die in your quest if you don't cease and desist. I see the truth of who you really are. You are nothing. Just a proud arrogant nothing.

23 And I will kill her children with death; and all the churches shall know that I am he which searcheth the reins and hearts: and I will give unto every one of you according to your works.

Here is proof that this is the heart chakra. The Truth will destroy you if you are a Jezebel Christian and everything that the lies in your heart propagated by your intimacy with demonic spirits. You will receive according to your works. If you do His works/move from His frequencies then your reward will be blessed. He searches your heart and tries your reigns.

Interestingly, *reins* in Hebrew means kidney. The kidney is responsible for blood pressure amongst many other things, keeping your body running smoothly. This chakras health depends on complete honesty and sincerity and unity with the Truth; a pure heart. Therefore, one must bring ones self before God daily and ask to be examined in the light of Truth in honesty.

24 But unto you I say, and unto the rest in Thyatira, as many as have not this doctrine, and which have not known the depths of Satan, as

they speak; I will put upon you none other burden.

The word Thyatira means 'continual sacrifice'. That means that those who remain in continual sacrifice of their flesh are *not* the ones who are following false teachings. These have not known the depths that devils can stoop to. They are honestly busy trying to please the Father in a corrupt and sick world. They may make mistakes and fall a thousand times, but their walk is sincere.

God knows that you are going through enough to continue to die daily as Paul did and so no other burden will he place on those who are continually sacrificing to the Lord.

25 But that which ye have *already* hold fast till I come.

If you don't let devils take away from your heart that which God has given you and you hold fast, God will reward you. You see the Truth and you hang on to it through continual sacrifice of self. David prayed to be cleansed from his secret faults. A heart can be a tricky thing.

26 And he that overcometh, and keepeth my works unto the end, to him will I give power over the nations:

If you overcome LF thoughts and ways and keep

the HF ones to the end of your life on earth God will give you the power to overcome nations. Why? The Truth will rule and reign through you. You will be an extension of Him, just as Jesus is now.

He showed you the right way to go and you held it at all cost to you personally. You did not sell out to what might have advantaged your flesh, you did not give in to taunts, pressure, mocking, and worldly reward. You didn't steal, you didn't hate, you didn't seek revenge, you obeyed Him in and from your heart. You kept your first love, you suffer bitter affliction, you rose above the world and it's ways and your heart has remained true and now you resisted the religious spirits of the day!

27 And he shall rule them with a rod of iron; as the vessels of a potter shall they be broken to shivers: even as I received of my Father.

Those who kept the Truth will rule with Jesus as He does and will be kings and priests. This happens now as it will in greater magnitude in the future.

28 And I will give him the morning star.

The Truth will be honored, lifted up for all to see. If you stand with the Truth, with the fact that it is wrong to gossip, wrong to love sin, wrong to glorify self, wrong to lust, and wrong to play god in God's name..... if you hold to the Truth you will rise with Truth for all to see. He will honor you with Himself.

29 He that hath an ear, let him hear what the Spirit saith unto the churches.

God's spirit, the center of your very own is saying that if you hear him in you, in your spirit, and don't do what the world is doing....no mocking, no slander, no abusing and using. If you do all that you know is right and good and hear Him in you then you will overcome the world and be with Him forever. This chakra point in the heart must be a place of *continual sacrifice.* The faithful are those who kept the Truth in their hearts till they died on earth.

This is where you bear your cross and where you learn to trust the Lord. It is a place with a weakness of listening to those who preach soothing sermons in disguise, messages from Jezebel telling you that it is okay to sin and be like the world, to have money, be important, special, powerful, wise, and evil. This is Jezebel's message to the church; many follow her unto death.

The pinker your aura, the more worldly your heart is, the greener it is means that your chakra is closer to God's heart and you have the gift of healing. Often people who have just received healing will have strong green in their auras.

Malfunctioning: Wicked heart, doubt, cowardice, unsure of right, self pity which is self love, possessive, jealous, shy, lonely, isolated, lack of empathy, bitter, critical, mean, cruel, and heartless. A heart centered on self and self gain. The mouth will give away the wicked heart. They never are sorry for anything and they secretly and sometimes openly hate others and are cruel and jealous.

Functioning: You should be able to hear your conscience easily and follow it. It is easy to be unselfish as you live for your Father in all that you do. You are developing into unity with Him becoming kind, patient, submissive to what is right and compassionate. The heart chakra is the one that gives us the sense of responsibility and purity and devotion. All our worries, doubts and fears are destroyed when the heart chakra is fully functional and in tune with God. A revelation of humilty would immensely help the heart chakra. Pride is its brutal enemy. This aspect of your spirit when functioning in tune with God's Spirit will express His heart as your own. You will have much compassion, tenderness, unconditional love, excellent equilibrium, rejection of evil, and well-being.

Physically the **Thyatira chakra** governs circulation and the circulatory system. Mentally it governs passion and you will live with great heart and by faith with great devotion if it is working properly.

Snapshot

4th Chakra : Thyatira/continual sacrifice

Color: greens...the lighter the green the healthier it is. Pink sometimes seems to overwhelm the green, meaning worldliness destroys the heart.

Location: heart

Sicknesses: heart disease, stroke, and heart area, and kidneys, high blood pressure, irregular heart beats, hole in the heart, etc,

Deadly sin that can block it: heart is wicked

Corresponding Armor: breastplate of righteousness

Divine Aura: girt about the paps with a golden girdle

(Your heart must become pure. This is a continual process of growth in Him. If you were like Him your heart would be golden and pure.)

5th Chakra>Sardis

This chakra or aspect of your spirit's energy governs such issues as self-expression and communication. Physically, Sardis governs communication, emotionally it governs independence of thought, mentally it governs fluent thought, and spiritually, it governs a sense of security in your thinking or heart.

Let's look at it through God's eyes:

1 And unto the angel of the church in Sardis write; These things saith he that hath the seven Spirits of God, and the seven stars; I know thy works, that thou hast a name that thou livest, and art dead.

Rev 3:1-6 (KJV)

Sardis means 'prince of joy'. If your mouth lines up with the Truth you are of a great joy to Him. He knows your works, and your name that your spirit is alive and your flesh is dead.

2 Be watchful, and strengthen the things which remain, that are ready to die: for I have not found thy works perfect before God.

I have yet to met a person with a perfect tongue. For out of the abundance of the heart, the mouth speaks and when the thought isn't coming out in words it is coming out in actions. However, the more your tongue aligns, the more you will be pleasing to God and the healthier this chakra will be.

3 Remember therefore how thou hast received and heard, and hold fast, and repent. If therefore thou shalt not watch, I will come on thee as a thief, and thou shalt not know what hour I will come upon thee.

How does one tame that tongue? The heart will make or break the tongue. Holding fast to what we know is right can only be done if our tongue complies. Watching is how you keep your tongue out of trouble and it is based upon receiving and hearing. Did we hear the Truth and hate it? Was it welcomed in us? Did we like it when we saw that we gossiped or that we slandered someone to teach them a lesson? Do we hate seeing our sin because we like the sin? If so how can we adjust our mouths to speak words of Truth? You must become the observer, not caught up in what is going on, but watching in open honesty.

4 Thou hast a few names even in Sardis which have not defiled their garments; and they shall walk with me in white: for they are worthy.

Lets talk about garments. What you wear signifies the state of your soul. I was thinking of how we wear our aura. A white aura means that your chakras are functioning properly. This is your white garment; a perfect chakra. It is high frequency vibrations being seen. The bride of Christ is dressed in white. You cannot fool God. Whoever is white will be the bride of Christ/joined to the Truth intimately forever. All your religious pretentious games will avail you nothing. God surely sees you just as you really are. How important then is it for us to see us as we really are so we can repent and align our hearts to His?

5 He that overcometh, the same shall be clothed in white raiment; and I will not blot out his name out of the book of life, but I will confess his name before my Father, and before his angels.

Is all the gossip in the world, all the judging, all the slander, all the ditching of government, all the mocking, condoning and condemning really worth it? How about your fake wonderful self? Your ego? Are you willing to trade Life with the Father for those stale morsels of death? No! May we all repent and be wearing clean garments. No words that are not His should be in our mouths.

6 He that hath an ear, let him hear what the Spirit saith unto the churches.

.

23 Whoso keepeth his mouth and his tongue keepeth his soul from troubles.

Prov 21:23 (KJV)

Malfunctioning: Eagerness to do evil is a good example of those who have no control over their tongues. Just think of how much sin there is right now in the world that begins and emanates from our lips. Lies and an inability to listen are signs that this chakra is blocked. Weight gain, fear of speaking, stuttering, poor rhythm, speaking just to be heard, are all signs that you don't have any control over your mouth. Harshness and lack of empathy create nasty words.

6 A fool's lips enter into contention, and his mouth calleth for strokes. 7 A fool's mouth *is* his destruction, and his lips *are* the snare of his soul.

Prov 18:6-7 (KJV)

Functioning: Your words will be His words, seasoned with salt and grace and timely. Only the truth will fall from your lips and even then they will only be spoken with understanding. You will be willing to admit to your faults verbally and your tongue would be speaking words of Truth. No guile will be found in your mouth. You may indeed have faults but you will be honest with God about what He shows you concerning them and seriously seeking to overcome them by dying to your flesh on a daily basis. God isn't going unload all of your wrong thinking at your feet and bash you in the head for being stupid. He will take His time helping you understand the error of your ways. As long as your heart knows no guile, your lips won't be speaking any. The Holy Spirit will lead you into all Truth. You may still be moving from wrong thinking in some areas but God has not shown you all of it yet. The difference, like I said, is that your heart is being honest with the Father and not trying to deceive Him.

Let's recap just in case you are missing the overall picture of growing up in Christ. A mature soul/spirit that has healthy auras will be as follows:

1st chakra>Have found the Truth/first desire
2nd chakra> Met bitter affliction for holding on to the Truth
3rd chakra>Risen above the affliction
4th chakra>Remained faithful and true to the Truth
5th chakra>The mouth is now in alignment and the aura is cleaner/lighter

4 These are they which were not defiled with women(demons); for they are virgins(pure). These are they which follow the Lamb(Truth) whithersoever he goeth. These were redeemed from among men, *being* the firstfruits unto God and to the Lamb. 5 And in their mouth was

found no guile: for they are without fault(s) before the throne of God.

Rev 14:4-5 (KJV)

Only a few make the cut of the 144,000, okay? Don't be discouraged if you see guile in your mouth. I've yet to met anyone who doesn't. Every person is exactly where they are at. Not where they imagine that they are, but exactly where they are. Just keep seeking the kingdom of heaven and thanking the Lord for His wondrous grace and realize that without the truth revealed to your soul you are DOOMED! Demons will capitalize upon your wrong thoughts, ride the frequency waves to your spirit and your life will bear their fruit. See the importance of separating from them. Every kind of sickness you can imagine is coming back on those dark waves and should you not resist them, your soul will pay the price and your candlestick will be removed. To be a part of the 144,000 you must honestly obey what He shows you and not move or speak against the Truth in your heart. It doesn't mean you are perfect, in that you have come into the full mind of Christ, but that you are perfectly living in all that you have received of Him thus far.

Guile means crafty or artful deception. This occurs because self is still much alive. You are trying to twist what God says just like you twist what other people say to get the meaning you want. Look at how you communicate. When you want to see yourself in a good light to be a good person so you can feel really good about yourself it means that you adore yourself. You cannot be good. It is impossible. A revelation on who you really are must occur before the deceit and guile will cease.

Snapshot

5th Chakra : Sardis/prince of joy

Color: light pale blue or turquoise. Dark blue indicates near death, light blue to white is spiritually seeking

Location: base of throat

Sicknesses: thyroid gland, weight gain, mouth, neck and throat areas

Deadly sin that can block it: eagerness to do evil/feet

Corresponding Armor: shield of faith

Divine Aura: voice as the sound of many waters

(You must have deep moral convictions before your mouth will align. Aligned your words would be holy and your voice would have meaning.)

6th Chakra>Philadelphia

What happens after the 5th chakra aligns in your spirit? This is where amazing things begin to happen and where you really begin to 'experience' God. This aspect or energy point is what many call your 3rd eye. It works in conjunction with your pineal gland which sits in the middle of your brain. It has to do with 'perceiving' or 'hearing' the Truth and with how you communicate spiritually.

This chakra point is very 'spiritual'. It is your eye into the spiritual world. If demonic spirits are ruling your chakras this eye will bring you uncontrollable demonic manifestations and can be used strongly in witchcraft. In the occult it is used for telepathy, astral projection, seeing spirits, remote viewing, drawing spirits, cursing others and used for harm. It is like your eyes and access to the spirit world.

It has a real function that it was designed to operate in and of. I believe the Word of Knowledge is one of the gifts that can manifest when this eye is opened. When it does open you may feel a strong pressure between your eyes and in the center of your forehead. It may be preceded by pressure in your occipital lobe which is located in your hind brain. On your forehead, it will feel like a thumb protruding outwards and a pressure may form over the top of your nose. This is a spiritual force you are feeling directly on your physical body. You can tell it is your own spirit because you can lift the pressure from your nose at will and the eye can be felt in its entirety, especially in cold weather. The third eye spans to the center of both eyes forming one large eye one in the center of your forehead.

Some people who have problems being demonically assaulted in their sleep, pulled from their bodies, and entered by astral projectors have taken my advice as to how to close the third eye. Just command it shut in Jesus name before you go to sleep. This has brought some people who have done this a fair amount of sleep!

My eye opened on its own. I did not even know that I had one. I knew nothing of chakras and such, but God, in His wondrous ways has led me where I am at today concerning these spiritual issues. The other chakras aligned through a series of repentances and the eye opened on its own.

I will include in the meditation a way to help develop your third eye the way I did and I'm glad that God is not afraid of spiritual things....after all He is the all Spirit God and all spirits are of Him so He's not uncomfortable with the aspects of our spirit.

Remember, spirits have functions just as our bodies have functions. To shy away from how your spirit works is a sure way to be a completely carnal christian and die in sin. Don't be like that. Embrace what God has given you and seek to be a good steward of all that he has blessed you with.

301

7 And to the angel of the church in Philadelphia write; These things saith he that is holy, he that is true, he that hath the key of David, he that openeth, and no man shutteth; and shutteth, and no man openeth;

Rev 3:7-13 (KJV)

God's Spirit is the only one that can open that eye up to function as it was meant to. If He shuts that door way, you will not be able to hear or see spiritually. You will be eternally blind and when you do use your 3rd eye it will be for evil and evil will come through it.

Philadelphia means 'brotherly love'. The key of David is referring to the fact that David was a man after God's own heart. This is the key to having the 3rd eye opened and functioning properly. Your heart must love the Truth and you must love your brother as yourself to use it properly. This is also the key to opening up yourself to revelations from God. You must hunger for the Truth to give to others. Your heart must be like your Fathers.

This chakra was not meant to open until your other ones were in line. If it opens before you are ready, you will get hurt and suffer because you will have no defense against the spirits that enter and assault you.

God is saying, "I am holy and true." He's showing you how you must be. Your mind must be in a continual process of renewing, the heart must be instructed and changing daily, and you must have some maturity in Him.

A pure desire to know the truth so you can help others will give you an open door into heaven. Those who come to God with selfish ambitions of money, fame, or power will find a door way open indeed, straight into the devil's lap! Nothing like the black fear of of the demonic realm entering your spirit to shake you in your boots! Waking up with scratches on you and bite marks, being pulled out of your body and chewed on, poltergeists, hauntings, and the list is long and lengthy as to the horrors that can come from that very dark world that hates all that is good.

They will not only torment your body, but begin to barrage you with every lustful and evil thought they can; feelings of hatred, strife, evil imaginations, nightmares, mental illnesses, and anger will begin to rule your life. This is the open doorway to the spiritual realm. Don't seek to open it and make it an ambition, instead seek to align your heart with God and He will open it when you are ready. Follow your Teacher and all will be well with you.

Brotherly love is spoken of by John. He who loves not knows not God for God is Love. This will be your character now, if your other chakras are working properly and from this brotherly love you will begin to perceive the things of God for He is Love. Sometimes the hardest thing to do for someone is the best thing for them. Be prepared and realize that real love is tough love. It always does what is good for you, not what brings itself the best reward. It isn't concerned with how many friends it has but the very lives and souls of others come before its own.

8 I know thy works: behold, I have set before thee an open door, and no man can shut it: for thou hast a little strength, and hast kept my word, and hast not denied my name.

When your works align with His, and you are doing His works....being patient, kind, generous, honest, humble...... when you stop the gossiping, slander, mocking, boasting, glorifying your fake self, speaking hateful words, being spiteful, and such and you begin to come in to the Light with true repentance, obedience to what you know is right, God will open up things to you and you will have this 'open' door and go from one glorious discovery to the next.

That door that is opened up to you that no person on earth can shut is your 3rd eye, His realm/HF. It is open because you had enough strength in your soul to see the truth and you kept it and did not deny who He is. As long as you stay in recognition of truth, even in a measure, this door will stay open to you! This is His promise to you. As long as you have some Love in your heart, hear some Truth, He will not shut the door on you. What a promise to all truth

304

seekers who trip over the shoelaces of sin. Thank you Jesus for grace!

9 Behold, I will make them of the synagogue of Satan, which say they are Jews, and are not, but do lie; behold, I will make them to come and worship before thy feet, and to know that I have loved thee.

Every person, every spirit, every creature that said they were of God but were not will bow at your feet one day! They will get to see it with their own eyes that God loves you because you love Him. So don't frustrate yourself and let your heart grow cold over the hypocrisy of others who say they are His and are not. He is the Truth and you loved Him even when the world, family, friends, all turned against you, saying that their wicked ways were of God and you didn't believe it and left them for what He showed you and you kept what you knew was right.

You knew the Truth and you did not deny Him, even though it cost you dearly on earth. You didn't join them in the gossip. You didn't play church games, you left when people started mocking others, you avoided evil, you kept your garments clean. In turn, He will not deny you! Even if all your ducks aren't in a row....... God will not shut the door on a sincere soul. Praise be to God! He is truly just!

10 Because thou hast kept the word of my patience, I also will keep thee from the hour of temptation, which shall come upon all the world, to try them that dwell upon the earth.

I have seen God keep this scripture in small measure. There are these 'hours' that come when you know that if He was not there to keep you from a temptation, that you would have no strength against it and would be swept away with the tide of this world. I have humbly watched Him not 'allow' me to enter certain situations that were to tempting for me. I have watched His hand keep me from those 'hours' my whole life. It is most humbling. I know that I could not have withstood and would have sinned had the situation not scooted around me or been plucked from my hands even against my will. He is a good Father.

Often when we desperately want something, God knows it is the worst thing that could happen to you. He will not allow it to be so. Money, for instance, everyone wants more and more of it, but God does what is best for your soul. If money were the answer to your salvation you'd be swimming in it. Instead He knows that you would indeed forget the Truth and live your life unto money and it will leave you one day soon when your body perishes and where will you be then having spent your life focused upon money? Trusting money with your whole heart is a quick way to die spiritually.

11 Behold, I come quickly: hold that fast which thou hast, that no man take thy crown.

He is coming. The Truth is coming to you. If you hold on tight to what you have, then no man can take away and rule your soul. The crown that you wear is the victory over this world 'in you' through receiving HF through your crown chakra! Once you've progressed this far down that road to heaven, your reward, your crown is direct access to the Divine Mind and revelations from which to live from. This is your 'crown' for having overcome what was destroying your spirit. Should you not 'hold fast' what was given you, the truths that were imparted, this crown, this 7th chakra will close again and your mind will become corrupt and death will come into your chakras.

When I describe to you what the 'crown' chakra is, you will understand the horrible loss you will have incurred should you be unable to 'hold fast'.

You lose the ability to live above the world when you let go of the truth and you fall for things like self pity, greed, lust, anger, and strife. Without Divine Revelations to move from you cannot overcome the world. You will fall and die. If you return to wrong thinking, like a dog does to its vomit, the world and death will once again become alive in you. This is what happens to those who have a wonderful experience with God, get born again, and then enter a 'dry' period. Have you noticed that they hate the mention of Jesus' name

307

once they've hit the dryness of their soul?

12 Him that overcometh will I make a pillar in the temple of my God, and he shall go no more out: and I will write upon him the name of my God, and the name of the city of my God, *which is* new Jerusalem, which cometh down out of heaven from my God: and *I will write upon him my new name.*

Whoever overcomes that which is not of God in them, only these people will partake of the Divine Mind. You cannot love, entertain and become a devil and have God's name written on you. It won't happen.

You have to become perfect in Him. And by that I mean that you have to be able to perfectly follow where He leads you. He is the Good Shepherd and will not lead his sheep up steep cliffs, through lava pits, and over glass shards. No, He leads you 'as' and where you are 'able' to follow. Should you decline to do what you should have done, that which His indwelling presence has shown you, should you love devil's ways over His— then you lose your crown.

Should you however, overcome the world in you, then you will become a permanent part of God Himself. Your name will be the name of God because you are truly bearing His name. You won't be coming and going from the Truth then a lie, then the truth, and then a lie.....double minded in all that you do. Instead, you will be at one with the Maker of the universe! You will be dwelling where God dwells and you will be doing whatever He does. Your name will be a new name...different from the one you were wearing and bearing. Perhaps you wore the name 'greed' or 'hate' or 'lust'?

This is more than my mind can even conceive! How much we give away for a crumb from the world. If people knew the price for their love of sin I don't think they would indulge with the same enthusiasm that we see today.

13 He that hath an ear, let him hear what the Spirit saith unto the churches.

Malfunctioning: Signs that you are not perceiving correctly are panic attacks, dementia, and many mental disorders due to overt demonic activity. Fear strikes the heart of a person who sees God and then denies Him, this is what happens when the third eye is opened through correction of the chakras and then the chakras become sick. The more Truth that you deny, the harder the attacks will be until you find yourself cowering down in your closet in full blown anxiety attacks.

Fear is for cowards and cowards are the ones who saw the Truth, yet refused it. It is in the refusal to see the Truth but a demand to know it that brings you to your knees. Hypocrites are people with

strong malfunctioning Philadelphia chakras. Being demonically attacked doesn't mean you are gifted in that area, it means that you have opened the doorway in ignorance and are now left with no 'strong man' to protect your spirit.

Functioning: If you would hear God's voice, the Word, and not plan and conceive mischief and deceit this chakra would be functioning properly. The whiter your aura, the more it is working. The darker the colors in the aura, the more worldly you are. The stronger and darker the colors the more out of alignment you are and the closer you are to death. A fully corrected aura will be light blue finally turning white and loose all color whereas a fully corrupt aura will be very dark blue, and turning black sometimes a week before death.

If the 6th chakra is functioning you will be able to perceive clearly and without struggle. This chakra is blocked by close mindedness or a willful desire to see only what benefits your goals and you. The more wicked your heart, the more demons you draw through this energy point into you.

Snapshot

6th Chakra : Philadelphia/brotherly love

Color: white/indigo blue, deep blue means worldliness, dark is close to complete death, black is death....usually within a week

Location: the brow/3rd eye/pineal gland

Sicknesses: dementia, panic attacks, Alzheimer, mental disorders

Deadly sin that can block it: planning mischief/conceiving

Corresponding Armor: eyes as a flame of fire

Divine Aura: helmet of salvation

(The third eye is responsible for spirit communication and how you perceive and affect other spirits and people. When this chakra is working properly you won't be taking directions from the dark world anymore through dark spirits but perceiving correctly and operating in the gifts you will be able to read other spirits and hear His voice directing you pertaining the lives of others which makes sense as it is supposed to operate from brotherly love. You will see through and by the fire of Truth. Helmets usually had a pace that come right over where the third eye is to protect it.)

7th Chakra>Laodicea

14 And unto the angel of the church of the Laodiceans write; These things saith the Amen, the faithful and true witness, the beginning of the creation of God;

The word Laodicea means"*people's opinions*" or "*people judged.*" Many theologians believe that these are separate meanings but it is because they do not understand what it really means. They think that God is speaking to a building full of people or a city and God is talking to your spirit man.

15 I know thy works, that thou art neither cold nor hot: I would thou wert cold or hot.

You have not judged yourself properly. If you had you'd be hot; on fire for the Truth. Your 'opinion' of yourself is not correct. Because you have not judged correctly having reached this spiritual threshold and shown you so much, He would rather you had never heard the Truth! You know why? Your punishment will now be severe!

16 So then because thou art lukewarm, and neither cold nor hot, I will spue thee out of my mouth.

Because you did not judge rightly, you knew the truth but you chose something else; your own opinions over His. The Truth will spew you out. This chakra point is the point of 'enlightenment'. This is the place in your spirit where He has revealed Himself to you strongly. If you look at and receive His revelations in your understanding and then go with 'your theories' over His Truth, your soul is toast!

17 Because thou sayest, I am rich, and increased with goods, and have need of nothing; and knowest not that thou art wretched, and miserable, and poor, and blind, and naked:

This is a really good description of the religious minded...those who spout holy words with absolutely no understanding. You will see them everywhere! Claiming to be prophetess and apostles yet they are the most hateful, nasty, people you can imagine doing everything for self glory. They look for every opportunity to get noticed. It is disgusting! They have no true idea of who God even is, they are just parrots, annoying disgusting things come out of their mouths as they speak for devils with glee. They stink up the place with their false teachings, pride, ego trips, and hypocrisy. They think they are holy and are not. They read the Word of God and refuse to obey it. They took the time to know the Truth and then promptly spat on Him. Even the world sees the hypocrisy and they laugh at you in your three piece suits and overstuffed opinions of yourself, driving your expensive cars and fleecing the sheep as if God were dead and not noticing.

You steal in the name of God, you justify your adultery with His word, you are a glutton and dare to take the pulpit and pretend that you know Him. You live lavishly, love money, and live just like the world.....hello!..... You are the world!.... and the world sees your game and you are mocking the Creator in your drunken stupor for self glory.

How many thousand books have been written with titles on making money and living well the 'Christian' way. I have seen Christian witches and Christian gays and Christian dating sights, and every 'Christian' scheme you can imagine. You might fool those who don't know God, but you will never fool those who do know Him nor will we ever join your sick twisted demented games. Your sins are in full view to those who love the Truth and if I can see you, you can be sure the Father does!

18 I counsel thee to buy of me gold tried in the fire, that thou mayest be rich; and white raiment, that thou mayest be clothed, and *that* the shame of thy nakedness do not appear; and anoint thine eyes with eyesalve, that thou mayest see.

God sees your filth. You will not fool anyone but those who are just like you. Be wise and repent before it is too late. The riches that you 'pretend' to have are fake and you are naked. Feel the shame of your love of the world, using God to climb your corporate ladder that you've established amongst the brotherhood. Anoint your eyes so you can see! Your chakra is not white.

19 As many as I love, I rebuke and chasten: be zealous therefore, and repent.

God does not wish any to perish and will chasten you for doing what you have done. You've taken Him into your being and then turned your back on Him. Be zealous and repent. Turn back to the first time you heard Him and remember your first love. This chakra is malfunctioning and will result in spiritual death if it does not repent and change and come into alignment with God.

20 Behold, I stand at the door, and knock: if any man hear my voice, and open the door, I will come in to him, and will sup with him, and he with me.

That door, that spiritual entry point is His mind and revelations being directly given to your own spirit and mind. He is at the door and knocking. His frequency is right there, ready to be accessed. If you will repent and turn to him fully He will come in and 'sup' with you. In other words, there will be a two way communication of HF.

However, if you are overcome by the world, in

love with fame, money, power, your body, and self centeredness, you will be rejected by God and He will not sit with you. There will be no 'one on one' for you with the Father. Is the world worth it? Are you really willing to step away from communion with God for your own ego? Do you really love the sound of devil's voices so much that you are willing to live with them forever? Stop playing your 'Jesus' game. Stop pretending that a lie is the truth. You are naked and all who love the Truth can see you.

21 To him that overcometh will I grant to sit with me in my throne, even as I also overcame, and am set down with my Father in his throne.

If you overcome this world, if you forsake everything that this world promises and seek only the Truth in all that you know and do, you will sit where Jesus sits in this world and the one to come. In other words you will come from the same place He does just as He comes from the same place God does. Your emotions, ways, and thoughts will be in alignment.

22 He that hath an ear, let him hear what the Spirit saith unto the churches.
Rev 3:14-22 (KJV)

God is talking to your entire spirit. You cannot be in an intimate knowing of yourself(the pretend you) and Him at the same time. Your spirit is either emitting LF or HF....there is no YouF. You cannot serve God and this world. If you believe/practice hate, greed, lust, envy, fulfillment of self, then guess what? If you are like the world, the world has overcome you. Your portion will be with the unbelievers...those who didn't believe the Truth either, those who practice their false thinking that they couldn't bear to let go of.

Do you know how people catch and eat wild monkeys? They put something shinny in a hole in a log, just big enough for the monkey to put his hand through but too small to pull the item out once he makes a fist and then the monkey is so greedy that he will die rather than let go of his shinny object! People can just walk up and whack the monkey in the head and eat him. This is you if you fall for the shinny lie of the devil. Don't be a monkey and die for nothing.

It won't matter what denomination you are of or how many times your butt warmed a pew! God isn't sending angels with counters to keep track of church attendance, okay? He's looking for sincere hearts who love to hear and follow the Truth! What did you do while you wore that body on earth? What were your frequencies/works? Did you do what you knew was right/HF? Did you seek the Truth or did you live according to your ego/LF?

To be really enlightened of God and to have His mind imparted to you. You have to have left the world behind. God will not give you revelations if you are you're own god because you are lovingly knocking on the wrong doors. He doesn't answer that door. If you serve yourself and not Him, He will not come and commune with you. You will not wear the 'crown'. You have to overcome the world/LF in you first!

I have seen so many people practice religion and miss God. They make everything about rituals and outward actions. Even the presence of God is all about something physical. Everyone wants the power of God. They 'brag' about being spiritual warriors! If you were spiritual, you wouldn't be bragging! That's an LF action. What they really want is to be God and they want God to help them accomplish their task and then get angry with Him for not showing up to serve them in their evil deed.

These kind are always the most fearful and hateful people. The ones who hurt others to further their pride. Exorcisms are all about them, their ministries are their prizes that 'prove' how no one is as amazing as them. They are walking contradictions and hypocrites. Their father the devil is just as they are, a murderer from the beginning, self-centered, fearful, cowardly, and a liar. Those who serve him behave just like him. They hate people without cause, are greedy, kill, and excuse it. They steal for the pleasure of it and destroy other people without remorse. They justify their sins and live arrogantly and only for selfish gain telling others that if you had 'faith' you could do it too. The liars, cowardly and unbelieving will be the first to warm the eternal fire and it will be a well deserved fate, one of which I hope mankind will be wise enough to avoid.

People cannot stomach Reality. They love their fabricated religions and pretense. If you want to make someone hate you just tell them the truth about themselves. Tell them what they already know is true about them and they will never speak to you again. Tell them to stop gossiping to you about someone and watch the phone slam down! Tell them they can't be your god and you aren't answering to them anymore. Tell them to quit trying to deceive you and quite lying to you. You want to make an enemy....tell him the truth. If speaking the Truth makes enemies does it mean that you lie a lot if you have many friends? It would behoove one to take note.

People who 'aspire' to take the throne of God are always looking for a way to become 'more spiritual'. It is sickening. Let your motives be pure. See that you are really nothing. All power is God's.

People who love themselves in his name often come to me for advice and it is pointless as they don't want to hear the Truth. What they are looking for is some way to get you to get God to agree with them. They think because I have so many experiences with God that I am great and they want to aspire to my greatness. Hello...I am nothing! What they really want me to do is find a way to help them live guilt free in their sins and be the wonderful great people that they always knew they were and this is just a fantasy folks. There is only One who is Great....and it isn't you or I. I guarantee it!

31 For if we would judge ourselves, we should not be judged.

1 Cor 11:31 (KJV)

People refuse to repent. They deny their faults and they continue loving their wrong thinking, yet they can pick out sin in everyone else without blinking and still continue to practice the same thing they just put down in another.....for this reason judgment will come to mankind. He's a hypocrite and a liar.

When the 7th Chakra is working properly a person will be humble and contrite and repentant. This person, the one to whom God 'really' talks to, is willing to see their faults, willing to admit the Truth, and they hunt their faults with a passion! They know that their faults separate them from God, so they hate them. Let me describe such a person to you.

If you see someone who has at least a nearly well spirit the first thing you will notice is that this person is not in love with the world or themselves. They don't care about the things you have or the things they have or don't have. This person also isn't interested in whether you like them or not nor do they get their 'feelings' hurt all the time. They don't want to hurt anyone and hate no one and feel no need to cling to anyone. They don't worry, fret, or agonize over this world—they are dead to it. Your opinions spoken to this person will matter little, for they don't serve people, only God. This person seeks the mind of God and wishes to know only those who know Him and their focus is to do all that they know is right and good. You don't have to worry about offending this person. Their heart and expectations are on God alone and they love you unconditionally which means that they will always do what is best for you even though you may not like it or them for doing it. Don't expect to win them over. There's nothing to win. They are good and kind to you because it is the right thing to do. They may often hurt your feelings, but it will be your own fault for not having died to your flesh and their words were ones you needed to hear to help you overcome your own flesh and the world. They don't seek large gatherings, or love the seats of notoriety. This world holds no 'magic' for them and they don't believe in the lust called 'love' by the world. They aren't interested in 'cultivating' people's friendships or maintaining any lofty ambitions or goals. They exist in and of Truth and deceit is their enemy, not people. They can tell the difference because without the goal of self gain, there is no point in hurting other people or using them.

Miracles are the norm. They live from the

providing hand of their Father and experience him daily. They don't look to anyone else for what they need as it would cause others to sin and have to play god in their lives. Their delight is in the law of God, not in or of this world and its ways and not in the tongues of devils.

They enjoy God's creation in the way He meant for it to be. Not in the 'having' of it but in knowing and experiencing of it as God's handiwork. They don't care if they die in body because they are already dead in flesh.....dead to lust, greed, selfishness, bribery, hate, anger, resentment, stealing, lying, cheating, and this world holds nothing for them. Their life is hid in Christ/Truth. All that they love, all that they live for, is God/Truth. This is the picture of a soul that loves God.

Let's be reasonable. You cannot take this world with you. If you spend your life for it where will you be when it is gone? This world is not just monetary gain but momentary gain. Love of this world as 'all that there is' is the root of all self centered and deceived lives. You believe that you can keep it forever and so you spend your life seeking that which is corrupt and your life ends in corruption.

Malfunctioning: Someone seeking knowledge for self advancement, intellectualism, and to know themselves better. They believe that the secret of life is in them and once they fully discover themselves, they will find it. They seek people to worship them, to affirm that they are indeed god. This kind does good deeds for reward. They put people on pedestals because they want one. This reaffirms to their hearts that pedestals exist.

The seventh chakra point is the place where enlightenment from above enters, but if you are of a wicked heart, God's mind won't be the mind leading you and 'enlightening' you someone else will instead. If your own lusts are at the bottom of all that you do, all that you do will be answered by devils and your so called enlightenment will be the blackest night and the darkest of thoughts.

I've seen those who gave themselves to the dark side. And woe unto those who open up, give, and seek the wrong kundalini.

Functioning: When all the other chakras are functioning properly, all the aspects of your spirit in alignment with the All Spirit God then you will be hot! Oh my gosh! There won't be enough brain space to hold the revelations. Paper won't help either! Wisdom will come while you eat, sleep, and work. God will open the floodgates of heaven upon you.

If some obstacle is facing me I don't try to move or fix it. I wait. Often by morning the information is just with me. God downloads it overnight as my life is His and I don't have problems, I have answers. God's ways are wondrous.

The warning that someone may steal your crown is referring to your ability to receive divine revelation via the top crown of your head. When this chakra is open, so is the kingdom of heaven to you. You will feel a prickling sensation that feels like little needles in the top of your scalp and the crown of your head. It will be very noticeable and tingly and sometimes pressure like someone is pushing down on your head with their finger.

Snapshot

7th Chakra : Laodicea/ people's opinions or people judged

Color: violet, turns light purple, to white when drawing nearer to God, darker when drawing nearer to demons or demons themselves sometimes are purple to black

Location: top or crown of the head

Sicknesses: demonic possession

Deadly sin that can block it: sowing discord among brethren, intentionally trying to destroy Truth in the lives of others...this is what demon possessed people do. They are a full extension of LF and cannot help but affect everyone they meet.

Corresponding Armor: Praying always with all prayer and supplication with all perseverance and supplication for all saints.

Divine Aura: His head and his hairs were white like wool

   (Interestingly, the crown chakra supplicates God. It transmits and receives enlightenment from above. You can feel the energy coming and going. The white head and hairs represent his pure aura.)

Recap

Can you tell the spiritual standing of a person just by looking at their aura and why can some people feel an aura instead of seeing it? Yes, both are possible because our spirits can sense, see, or perceive other people's auras or energies and what is or isn't correct in it.

This is the 'creepy' feeling we get a lot of times when we meet people or for the instant feeling of what some call 'kindred spirits'. Is it because the auras are nearly identical and bring us comfort? Learn to ask questions of God and not require an answer to come immediately. Learn to stay in a state of wonderment in humility and wait for God to come and share with you.

Aura's.....the colors....is this also how demons can can tell your weaknesses? Is the doorway a bio-electric frequency that can be felt and seen? Are spirits entering because of our own sin? Do they see, feel, and perceive it the same way you are sensing it in others, only in a clearer more defined way? If this is true they do not really have to enter to know you and read you. Perhaps when we resist them, they never even actually enter. I have so many questions that are yet to be answered.

Sifting, is this the process of analyzing

someone's aura, faults, and chakras?

And the Lord said, Simon, Simon, behold, Satan hath desired *to have* you, that he may sift *you* as wheat: 32 But I have prayed for thee, that thy faith fail not: and when thou art converted, strengthen thy brethren.

Luke 22:31-32 (KJV)

Can we protect others from entry? When we pray for one another are we sending them our positive frequencies and strengthening them? We can see the difference positive thoughts have over negative ones in scientific experiments. Surely the same affect applies to our bodies and souls.

If the Chakra is functioning properly, as God intended, or at least within a healthy range of it are demons unable to enter and if so this would explain why a change of heart and soul, called repentance, can set things aright and bring immediate deliverance that people experience?

31 Then said Jesus to those Jews which believed on him, If ye continue in my word, *then* are ye my disciples indeed; 32 And ye shall know the truth, and the truth shall make you free.

John 8:31-33 (KJV)

One fact I'd like to point out here that sin is sin and truth is truth no matter what religion you claim you are or where you come from. Stealing is stealing in any language and so is doubting what is right, that is to say, what your heart knows is right even without a word being spoken. Truth doesn't need our petty words attached to it. It is God and stands for itself and by itself and the stars bear witness of Him. They move in their orbits and obey in perfect order. He calls them all by name and needs the counsel of no one nor does He need their help. The Truth is who He is and He is unchanging. What He does, stands, whether we comprehend it or not. Glory to His holy sacred name.

We have seven spiritual components or chakras, an aura, and our spirit is the church of God; the place where God resides. Our auras are either in or out of alignment with God's Spirits which has seven aspects. When our bodies get sick it is because these chakras are not functioning properly as God intended. All living organisms get their nourishment from an outside source and then the nourishment is turned into food within the organism. Our spirits are the same way and we are not self existent, that is to say, independent from the true Light. The only Light that can exist in us is the Light of Truth and it is Him in you that brings life to your body, spirit, and soul.

Your chakra is your spirit and your spirit is your chakra and it is designed to receive, assimilate, and express God's Spirit. This is your true self. There are high and low frequencies. You are emitting either one or the other in every thought you think and every emotion you move from.

.Eleven

How the Law of Attraction Really Works:

Every thought has a frequency.....

This chapter is somewhat of a recap but on a more in-depth level. It is imperative for you to understand that you are a product of your own thinking and emotions. You have made you who you are today. Every thought and emotion you moved from brought you an effect. These thoughts and emotions came about from a series of events in your life. Therefore society, parents, culture, education, and such things have much to do with who we are but the final decision became one of the heart when each and every thought was presented to us by other people. We(our bodies) have become our hearts/spirits.

There are a lot of scams out there and one of the biggest is the Law of Attraction. The reason I call it a scam is because you cannot follow it as it is designed or be successful at it; actually, it is impossible. Bear with me and I will show you why this is true.

Man, does not exist apart from God. Man is a part of God as God is all and in all. Therefore, man is designed to function by the Creator in only a specific way. Only by moving within the designs of the Creator can He find blessings. I'm going to show you how to live in and of God's hand so you can be blessed in all that you do. I also want you to understand that cursings and things like accidents don't come upon you 'accidentally'. We are bringing them to us by what we do and don't do, think and don't think. The thoughts and emotions behind the scene in your life are like tiny emitters calling into action spirits who create your answers. One day you will go to be with the one you emitted/loved the most.

There are a 'few' cases where a person is a victim of circumstance. One example is a true widow or an orphan and they are few compared to the many lives that this world has seen come and go. Don't be saddened if you realize that you are the creator of your own problems, instead be happy because it means that you will soon see a way to overcome them all. This way can only be found by those who love the Truth. It is the 'high-way' of God.

Fact # 1   Energy/Spirit is the source of all matter

This is God, the Divine Mind/Spirit. Everything you see originated from Spirit *and still does today.* He is all and in all and all power/energy is His and is Him. He is everywhere at once, all inclusive, and nothing exists outside of Him. There are 'no' other powers. The energies that be are 'ordained' by Him.

Everything you see is spirit vibrations. God cannot be less than He is or added to as He is all. Therefore creation is in Him and nothing of Him is ever lost.

Spirit creates matter. Spirit is Energy. Energy is cause. Matter is effect. Matter is a lower energy and can effect other matter but cannot change Spirit. Notice that he created 'dominions, powers, principalities'. These are have become in essence 'the rules' of life.

7 I form the light, and create darkness: I make peace, and create evil: I the LORD do all these *things*.

Isaiah 45:6-7 (KJV)

The spiritual laws that God created also include the cause and effect of evil. He created evil. It is much like His shadow. It is of Him but He is not in it. His character traits are not in His shadow, neither is His heart or His mind. A shadow is void of understanding, love, kindness, or empathy. It is cold, dark, empty, and not able to exist on its own.

Fact #2: Every Thought Has a Frequency

Science has proven that every thought has a frequency. Your body itself emits energy waves. You can feel the heat coming from your body. It can be measured and we use such technology such as brain entrainment today in science to help heal people.

When you move from an emotion or a thought that is outside of God's own thoughts and ways, you begin to emit a low frequency. This frequency is then picked up in the demonic or lower realm where those who aren't saved abide. Ghosts emit low frequencies. Again, you can purchase the meters from many places nowadays. Lower frequencies are a sign that you are headed towards death.

If you move from a high frequency thoughts and emotions, (which is any thought or emotion that is of God), then God responds to your thoughts and emotions, moving seamlessly through your life as you become at one with Him. Eventually those who emit high frequencies will enter heaven. First in spirit, then in flesh(glorified or transformed).

Your spirit has seven high energies or levels of frequencies that it emits and seven ranges of low frequencies. You are being recorded in heaven/God's data base/Mind. What you emit in your life time is written down and kept on record for judgment day should you not make the first cut and become one of the first-fruits. God is going to let everyone know how they did. He is fair and just and perfect.

Fact #3   Like Frequencies Respond to Like Frequencies

The bible says that if you cast your bread on the water, it comes back to you. This means that what you send out returns, just like it is. If you send out a low frequency thought (corrupt signal), it will return to you cursed or corrupt...just like you sent it out. Everything you do will be cursed if you move from low frequency thoughts.

21 Jesus answered and said unto them, Verily I say unto you, If ye have faith, and doubt not, ye shall not only do this *which is done* to the fig tree, but also if ye shall say unto this mountain, Be thou removed, and be thou cast into the sea; it shall be done. 22 And all things, whatsoever ye shall ask in prayer, believing, ye shall receive.
$$\text{Matt 21:21-22 (KJV)}$$

It is 'impossible' for you to not receive the good that you ask for from God if you move from deep moral convictions in what you seek. You are creating your own future by the thoughts and emotions you move from. God doesn't hear or 'respond' to low frequency vibrations with blessings. He won't listen to selfish or evil requests and encourage you into eternal oblivion.

12 Verily, verily, I say unto you, He that believeth on me, the works that I do shall he do also; and greater *works* than these shall he do; because I go unto my Father.

13 And whatsoever ye shall ask in my name, that will I do, that the Father may be glorified in the Son. **14** If ye shall ask any thing in my name, I will do *it*.

John 14:12-14 (KJV)

Here is the secret. You have to move from His revelation, emotions, and thoughts in you. You hear and receive from the spirit that you come from. Ask from the correct place in your heart, and then stand upon what you have been shown and it 'will' come to pass. While that seems vague right now, I will expound upon it in a way that hopefully will help you understand. Basically, where people miss it is that they have very little divine revelation to move from but begin their journeys in life from self discovery instead of Truth discovery. Their religions are based upon what others have been shown as they are not willing to go through the fire of repentance to hear the Truth in their hearts for themselves. Just like the Israelis they would rather Moses go to the top of the mountain and talk to God than feel their own smallness. Everything is external to them. Their faith becomes that of the pastor or the denomination that they claim they follow. In the end, they are robbed, lifeless, and going to hell 'hoping' they are saved. They are not.

If you move from lusts (corrupt desires based on selfish ambition), instead of divine revelations and the heart of God, God will not be manifest in your life. He will not support a demonic mind or any thought or way that is not correct. All thoughts and emotions that come from your lusts are low frequency vibrations and are picked up by demons. They will come and you get exactly what you wanted. You may even thank the Lord for what you prayed for and He is not the one who brought you your answer. The moment you moved upon a demonic/evil thought or an emotion, from then on what you will receive into your life will be cursed.

7 Ask, and it shall be given you; seek, and ye shall find; knock, and it shall be opened unto you:

8 For every one that asketh receiveth; and he that seeketh findeth; and to him that knocketh it shall be opened.
Matt 7:7-8 (KJV)

Everyone that asks (that's good and bad sources, high and low frequency transmissions) receives back. Whatever you seek, you find. This is the law of God and why no person will have ought to say on judgment day. Whatever door/frequency you are knocking on, that will be the door that opens and you will get 'exactly' what you want. Only the door of God, however, will return with blessings attached to it. Demons will answer all negative thoughts, wishes, and emotions. You may well get that money or that babe, but it will be cursed from one end to the other!

Imagine yourself standing in a room; this room is your mind and heart. You have just two doors exiting. One door is labeled high frequency the other low frequency. Every time you move from an emotion or a thought that isn't in the high frequency range the low frequency door pops open and in comes the dead and all their friends stinking up the place with their corpses. They come bearing gifts for you. A hot woman with aids, children you'll never get to enjoy, a house you'll never have time to live in and the list is long and lengthy. You start to die spiritually and become like them and the room starts to darken as death becomes you. The only way to get rid of them is to open the other door and let the Light in. This door can only be opened by a correct thought, desire, or emotion standing foremost in your life. If you so much as even wish for the truth, this door will respond to you. This is what you are facing in real life. Every door that stays open for any length of time will produce fruit in your life. One produces blessings and the other cursings. I have noticed that in major things like relationships and things of this nature that 2 years seems to be a normal waiting period for the thought to come to pass. I'm sure there are many variable times and ways as God is just and fair and wishes that none would perish.

If you move from wrong emotions and thoughts you may well get the money you lusted for, but it will leave you or you will be too busy to enjoy it. You may get that woman you wanted, but she will rule over you. You may get those children you always dreamed of but they will be sick, or hate you, or be taken away by that woman you had to have for 'yourself'. Every single thing in your life that turned out badly, failed, or disappointed you was because you moved from a wrong place in your heart to attain it. Look back and be honest and you will see how your own thoughts have brought you to where you are today. You made life all about you, were entirely selfish, and those were low frequency thoughts and emotions. You left the devils door wide open. You become your friends! Whose company did you keep? Whose company are you holding as we speak? Real life company will tell you clearly what spirit you entertain. For all who love the Truth will not seek the company of fools and all fools hate the wise for wisdom exposes treachery.

2 Ye lust, and have not: ye kill, and desire to have, and cannot obtain: ye fight and war, yet ye have not, because ye ask not.

3 Ye ask, and receive not, because ye ask amiss, that ye may consume *it* upon your lusts.

James 4:1-3 (KJV)

I've had dreams where I drink and drink and can never quench my thirst and awoke thirsty. This is a lot like your flesh. You will never get what you really need because you are asking amiss. You feel the nakedness of your soul and instead of coming to God to cover your naked spirit you go the shopping mall and spend all the money you don't have(credit cards.) A new car isn't the answer to your heart not feeling like it is good enough. The money you killed yourself obtaining won't bring you happiness. The hot woman won't make you more of a man. The kids won't give you real purpose in life. And your dog following you around doesn't mean that you are worthy to be worshiped. You are asking amiss by seeking your answers from a wrong place in your heart and you aren't receiving because you are moving from lusts instead of divine revelations.

Fact #4   Creation Powers are Within Yourself

God has designed this world to express us. We are making it like us. He put creation powers inside of each and every person. Every time you move from a right place in your heart the angels move in accordance to your thoughts and bring to you your desires.

You cannot move from corrupt thoughts, lusts, wrong emotions, a desire to acquire for self gain and dwell in the blessings of the Creator. You may bring

338

what you desire into being but it will come to you cursed.

God expects you to move and live from faith. Faith means 'moral convictions'. Every time you move from what you know is right the angel's respond. If your convictions are deep and really strong the frequency is also strong.

God's ears are only open to the prayers of the righteous. This means that he is aware of the low frequency thoughts and ways, but he doesn't answer them with His presence and His angels. He lets his evil angels and demons come to the aid the low vibrations. This is His answer to every disobedient child.

Fact #5 Unstable Wishing/Frequencies Will Get You Nowhere

The way to receiving from God is clearly written in the bible. Here are the steps.

4 But let patience have *her* perfect work, that ye may be perfect and entire, wanting nothing.

If you have the correct thought concerning whatever is facing you then you have the correct frequency to move from. Now you are to continue in what you know is right. You are to wait patiently and not doubt what you know is right. In your patience you possess your soul. No demon is in charge. Your works will be perfect and your spirit frequency will be entire and without corruption.

5 if you lack wisdom, let him ask of God, that giveth to all *men* liberally, and upbraideth not; and it shall be given him.

If you don't have the spiritual revelation/high frequency you need to move on so you can wait for your reward to come, all you need to do is ask the Father for it. He gives to all men liberally without rebuking them. Anyone who wants the truth will get it.

6 But let him ask in faith, nothing wavering. For he that wavereth is like a wave of the sea driven with the wind and tossed.

When you ask for it you have to move from faith. He only hears high frequency, remember? If you fearfully or in self pity cry out for wisdom, you are sending out 'low frequencies'. He only hears His children and answers their prayers. His children are high frequency emitters, okay? You have to move from faith which is a deep inner conviction that God will keep his Word and the revelation will come to you. Every person has a measure of faith in them. Once you receive the revelation stand fast. It will be the correct thought to think. You are to keep that thought foremost concerning your situation and in time you will be rewarded. The angels will bring you the answer to your frequency.

7 For let not that man think that he shall receive any thing of the Lord.

A person that has the truth, drops it, has it again then changes his mind and can't decide what to do is like a broken emitter. The reason you waver is that your heart is not fully submitted to God. You are trying to discern what benefits you and playing the field. Your instability will cost you as your future will be a waste of time. Start your journey by diligently searching your heart and you will be rewarded for it.

8 A double minded man *is* unstable in all his ways.
James 1:3-8 (KJV)

3 Thou wilt keep him in perfect peace, whose mind is stayed on thee: because he trusteth in thee.   **Isaiah 26:3 (KJV)**

Your convictions need to be deep. Your mind must be able to not wander. Fixations, dreams, evil imaginations and the ego (your pretend amazing self) are all great enemies of Truth. Your faith, what you know is right, must be in the Truth.

Fact#6 God supplies according to the Goodness of His Heart

When you are content with what the Father gives you and you aren't in danger of sinning against him with your things, then God can give you more things. If you swell up in pride and think that it is because of your goodness, wisdom, or power that you have what you have, then this will cause you to stumble. God's priority is our souls, not our flesh. He doesn't exist to bolster your ego and serve your imaginary self. As long as a person puts their flesh above their soul, they will have trouble in the flesh.

6 **But godliness with contentment is great gain.**

7 **For we brought nothing into *this* world, *and it is* certain we can carry nothing out.**

8 **And having food and raiment let us be therewith content.**

9 **But they that will be rich fall into temptation and a snare, and *into* many foolish and hurtful lusts, which drown men in destruction and perdition.**

10 **For the love of money is the root of all evil: which while some coveted after, they have erred from the faith, and pierced themselves through with many sorrows.**

1 Tim 6:6-10 (KJV)

342

You will find once your heart is getting what it needs from God that you won't want all those things that people use to try to be happy. You won't be living extendedly through your things. You won't have to have a big car to prove you are amazing. Diamonds are really just pretty rocks and they have no value to you beyond that nor do you wish to covet them and horde them. Reality will give you all things that you thought you had lost or not attained. A person who lives within the Truth is a person who is complete— lacking nothing.

It has been my experience that God loves to give me things and surprises me all the time, however, I would never consider the things the source of my joy but rather, like a token of love from my Father. All things, even those that appear to be in my possession are really His and one must always remember that everything is the Lord's.

It is okay to not have things. People just don't know that anymore. Happiness does not consist in the material possessions that one has. If it did then the rich would never know sorrow. Money without godliness brings much sorrow and the pursuit of it will destroy your heart and life.

God will look at your heart and answer the wishes and prayers that come from a right place. He does so in His timing, His way. God loves you and will always do what is best for you. Often, what we wish for would be the worst thing for us and God, in His great love, makes all things work out for good for those who are His. All creation is being shaped and mentored by Him. Some will find Him in this life and some the next. Sadly, some will never know Him.

Examples of Frequencies:

Emotions/Frequencies that are low:

Any thought that comes from greed, lust, envy, bitterness, anger, resentment, jealousy, hatred, strife, variance, debate, perversion, unnatural affections, selfish or self centered actions or thoughts, cruelty, spiteful, vengeful, hateful or hurtful thoughts or ways, impatience, hot temper, spiteful, proud, arrogant, self advantageous actions, lies, etc.

Emotions/Frequencies that are High:

Patient thoughts, kind, loving, faithful to what it knows is right, waits on the Lord (only God has what it needs), endures mockery and persecutions (knowing its reward is of the Lord), not greedy (God provides for it), not hateful (no reason to hate anyone), gentle, enduring, faithful, loving, patient, unmovable, does what is best for others, humble, and speaks the truth, etc.

Two examples to draw from:

a. A man wants money. He can just see how everyone will be so impressed by his life once he has the 'money'. Everyone will want to be like him and be his friend; he will be so adored, so powerful. Girls will very likely throw themselves at him and he may or may not take advantage of them; he loves that he'll have to decide. He envisions himself as being truly happy the day he finally gets the 'money'. He is moved by greed and selfish ambition. Remember, the stronger and deeper the desires the stronger and more perverse the answer will return.

The money finally seems to come in. He's got a great job and investments to boot. He lauds himself for his wisdom and it seems it is all coming true. He truly is amazing, just as he had always suspected. He's reassured in his own heart and preaches it loudly that you 'just have to follow your dreams.' He soon realizes that he can't stop working or his position will be in jeopardy. His work is stressful and his health begins to decline. He can't keep a woman because she wants all of his attention, which the business demands, and kids are out of the question....who has time for them? He begins striving hard to make up for the loss of both, promising himself he'll slow down when he gets enough ahead. Investments start backfiring and he tries to ease the stress with a few hot babes on the side every now and again, to prove to his ego that

345

he's still 'the man'. Time flies, he begins to bald. Panicking he gets married before its too late. All this stress is setting him up for death as he moves further and further away from God/Truth. He has a mild stroke. The doctor tells him to quit his job, but he can't. His money owns him. What is he without it? His woman, who sees him as a god, would surely leave him. Did he really get the money or did the money get him? To top it all off one of the hot babes is pregnant and it's twins! Now he's going to pay child support, will probably loose his wife, and 'he can't stop working' for two reasons. One, he is defined by his position and to lose his position is to lose his life. Two, all the people in his life were pulled in by his own desire to be noticed in the position that he has. If he loses that position, he knows that they will go away too. The money owns his soul both while living and surely in death. Does this sound like Hollywood to you? No wonder they have so many suicides and traumas.

b. A man needs money. He has bills to pay. He knows in his heart that money is just paper and all creation is God's. He wants to make his life count, do something good with it. He decides to do what his heart loves— gardening. "I will sell seeds that aren't genetically altered", he thinks to himself. He envisions all the people of the world who open his packs of seeds and grow good healthy food and vegetables that don't make them sick. He sees them feeding their families for generations to come. His

346

mind says, "It doesn't matter how much money I make at it, as long as it will pay the bills." Believing in the dream that is good, he gets to work with all his heart. He ambitiously does the good that his heart envisions.

His business grows despite the bad economy. His heart on this issue is good, therefore his work is before the Lord. This is a true story. I choose not to mention the name but his business is abounding and one of the best seed companies out there offering all heirloom seeds. He's also been blessed with a lovely wife and child and many who truly enjoy his company and his business. They are becoming the largest seed company of its kind holding many possessions. They are blessed. He enjoys his life. Eating his healthy veggies will prolong his days upon the earth and many lives will be blessed through his life/ministry. His message is one of living beyond your self for what is right.

Look at your own life for the testimony. Every time you moved from an emotion that was not right, what became of it? How many things have you done in anger or greed that resulted in disaster? Your lusts — they enslave you. Your desires and wishes set you up for a life time of servitude. Even your coffee owns you. Without it you are a mess!

It is impossible for good to come from evil unless it is the means whereby you learn the difference between right and wrong, finding salvation.

11 My son, despise not the chastening of the LORD; neither be weary of his correction: 12 For whom the LORD loveth he correcteth; even as a father the son *in whom* he delighteth.

Prov 3:10-12 (KJV)

Only when evil becomes a lesson does evil bless our lives. This is why all things work together for them that love good. Evil will merely become a lesson of what 'not' to do. How many people live as if God was going to bless them for doing evil? They actually believe in their hearts that sinning is a good thing to do and that it will bless them. It is impossible. Evil will overcome all who are evil at heart because they are emitting low frequencies. You are creating your future. If you dwell in your past your future frequencies become your past frequencies which is why you have to forgive others to enter heaven. All who do not and who dwell upon the low frequencies, these will die.

Your wishes are your prayers. What are you wishing for? All fears will be answered as fear is a low frequency and what you fear will come upon you. You are calling it to you. Job's fear came to him. Do you see now why it is so important to have your mind renewed? All who are reborn unto high frequencies are the church of God or the place God's Spirit dwells and all who vibrate high wear white(auras) and are the bride of Christ. The rapture occurs in the 'air'. This is where all who are wearing white will meet the Lord/Truth at and be with Him forever. Are you willing to see your faults so you can leave them behind to be with Christ? Or do you love your wrong thinking more than you do Life itself?

Twelve

The Meditation:

Sitting in the Presence of God.....

Now, what I want to show you is that you can sit in God's presence in a special way to help repair your chakras/frequencies and in doing so your garments(aura) will become white as snow. You see now why it is so important to make sure that you are thinking the right thoughts and coming from the right emotions. So now it is time to come to God in a serious way.

Please finish reading this chapter and then get the meditation audio download from my website to do the meditation properly. After you get the hang of it, you can do it on your own easily. Make the commitment to meditate regularly 'before' you begin meditating because that is what will make the difference between success and failure.

I am so thankful to the Father for showing me how to do this. I can see why David meditated all the time and I understand now how he was able to write much from God's Divine Mind. The meditation allowed him to separate from self to hear clearly.

This is not what the church calls soaking as they use all kinds of music and emotional stimuli. This will create deeper fixations and make you more religious and obedient to people and religion. Although soaking works wonders for the finances of modern Churchianity, lining the pockets of the proud men who love to be worshiped in God's name, I would like you to actually get to know God rather than becoming more hypnotically attached to misguided thoughts. Soaking will result in an emotional high that feels good, but so does sex, new shoes, and gooey chocolate. It doesn't mean that you've improved spiritually. To improve spiritually one must go through repentance. This is a process whereby one leaves the dark by coming into the Light. You don't grow close to God by shaking, quaking, shouting, feeling chills, falling over, fixating on images in your mind or such nonsense. Again, your closeness to God comes by a process called 'repentance' whereby a soul leaves false ways, emotions, and thoughts for correct ones. Salvation is a matter of the heart, not the flesh.

The true test of whether you met with God has to do with one question, 'do you have more truth in your heart?' God is Truth, and if you have just spent some time with Him, you will have some truth opened up to you. If you are into 'religion' (the act whereby one discovers themselves as god in God's name) sitting still with the Truth will be your worst nightmare!

"Please! Don't turn on the light!", the hypocrites scream as they cover their filthy garments and stinking pride by the folds of the dark night, "we only want to see and worship ourselves, not the Truth! Quick....make more noise and act religious so no one will notice how much we love sin!"

This meditation is for sincere Truth seekers only! One must be able to discern and focus upon the voices in the Spirit realm and it is imperative to be able to hear and give one's full attention to the Father. The Father is Reality. By staying in Reality and not being pulled away into a dream or fantasy you will be sitting directly in His presence and able to perceive Him. It is that simple.

48 Be ye therefore perfect, even as your Father which is in heaven is perfect.
Matt 5:48 (KJV)

I now understand this verse and what it means by 'perfection'. If you live perfectly obedient to everything His Spirit is revealing to yours, you are indeed the 'perfect'. God really does expect you to be perfect and you are most certainly able to do it.

Remember, if any of your seven entry points becomes fully blocked you will die quickly; slowly if partially blocked. The energy behind rejuvenation will be cut off and demons and death will enter where life was meant to be. This is how and why

352

sin/wrong thinking acted on is the main cause for sickness and why healing comes to us via the cross. This comes to you by your own frequencies that you emitted. This is what must change— the heart.

Imagine if you would seven vital tubes or veins of blood pumping directly from God into your body. Each vein keeps a portion of your body alive, your body having seven areas of life all independent yet reliant on the other for survival. Imagine now if one of these vital sources of blood were to become even partially blocked. That area of your body would slowly disintegrate until it finally fails. Because all the other parts need it to survive, your body begins to shut down, death is imminent. Unless the blockages are removed you will soon die. When an illness goes into remission it is because some repentance took place and the blockages are lessened.

Sin is not a magical substance that falls on you at birth. It is a state of consciousness that comes to you the moment you are conceived in the womb because we are born into a low frequency world, and emit them from birth; we are born in sin. Babies are birthed forth with characters already in place and our flesh rules us from the first hunger pangs to the first wet diaper. Every mother already knows somewhat of her babies character before it is born; just ask her. Where is the road back to our Creator? It can only come through seeing the Truth, repenting, and making the Truth that which rules your life.

The meditation is a process that allows you to quiet down, pull away from distractions, and hear and observe your own spirit in the light of Reality. If your spirit were to align perfectly I believe that you would simply not be here anymore— like Enoch. However, the closer you align with God, the healthier you will be and every day you are either growing and advancing in what is true or what is not true. If a spirit does not have the likeness of the Son of man in the midst of it, it will not be saved upon death of the body. Only His indwelling presence redeems us. Our core must be His Light in us.

I've had people argue that they've seen a lot of healthy wicked people and I would say to you, "come back and check on those healthy wicked people in a few years and tell me how they are doing." I know that God's spiritual laws cannot be avoided or evaded. His mercy endures forever but He is Justice and He has spiritual laws that are in effect and are no respecter of persons. Man reaps what he sows. There is no need for us to punish anyone. God is not dead. Evil has its reward. Good also has a reward. We only have two roads to travel, folks.....one is called 'Blessings' the other 'Cursings'.

In the bible, the Lord's prayer shortly follows the scripture expressing that we should be perfect as He is perfect and if really prayed according to the Lord's prayer with pure intent it will help align your chakras which is also why many use it to ward off evil because it does if prayed in earnest and will help to align your spirit with God's. Your enemy is one that lies within you. Therefore, the battlefield is within and seeing it is such let's begin with the meditation positions that I have found the most helpful. I suggest, if you can, do it three times a day or at least once in the morning and once at night. I want you to forget what you've been taught about prayer for the moment. Churchanity doesn't know what it is talking about. If it did, all those chanting and ranting prayers would have changed the world instead of making it worse. I hope that many people become free from Churchianity to lead real lives of Truth and set the world ablaze with the Light of God. If you actually go back to the times when you really knew that God heard you you'll see that a word was never spoken but your heart cried out in deep contrition and earnest desire to hear the Truth. You cannot hear God through earthly desires.

(Hopefully, by the time this is published, there will be a free guide on my website and e-book but if not, check back soon at **http://www.breadandwineministries.org** *as I plan to do this for people to help restore them to health and wellness. I also hope to eventually offer prayer cabins on my property to use for free and hold classes on how to meditate and should one need a deliverance; that would also be available to help them get well and live healthier lives.)*

The correct position in meditating is key because

you do not want to fall asleep yet you want your chakra points to align. You cannot align your own chakras by force, as that is pride...a negative thought, but what you can do is access the Father in you and He will do it. Sleep is your biggest temptation and danger. Most people are already in a sleep state or a hypnotic state and I don't want to encourage anyone to continue or deepen it. When you are really tired, your mind tends to wander anyway and I want you to 'watch and pray' not 'forget and dream'.

Many and most of the meditations you see are merely foolish affirmations and movement of a wrong or negative energy source this results in creating more problems than answers. Some meditations that I came across were designed to give demonic spirits full possession of you even satanist recognize its advantages and use the kundalini meditation exercises due to the easy access to demonic spirits. The Roy Master's meditation is good and certainly worth doing but I have found a way I like better; a way that ministers to your entire spirit man.

In order to meditate properly you must begin with the right motives. You must do the meditation simply because you want the truth in your life. You want God's mind to move from and to live unto His mind instead of demons. All your illnesses and problems must come second to that and you must be willing to move at God's pace and not have some other agenda. Only when you die to this world(low frequencies) can you be well in it.

When a person attempts to 'fix' themselves, even that action can be tainted with pride and any meditation will not work in its fullness because all you will be doing is drawing a demonic spirit of pride to aid you in knowing yourself as something you are not....hence delusions of grandeur will be all you that you end up knowing and you will experience a wonderful daydream about how real all your deceptions are to you and you will become hypnotically attached to the meditation and use it to get emotional relief. I don't want that to happen to you. If that's all you want, by all means try soaking.

To really reach perfection or oneness with Truth, you have to honestly come into the Light where the Truth is at. Therefore, you cannot set any preconceived goals for yourself like I will be healed, smart, or happy, etc. You must come into the presence of God in sincerity of finding Him, not hoping to know or see yourself in a better light or find out all your wonderful qualities that make you think you are amazing, special, and worthy. If you are into 'self' discovery you aren't into 'God' discovery. See, what people do not understand is that you are not who you think you are and then you live out of deception and lies and die. Even the voices that you think are yours, are not. You are the observer. This other person that calls itself 'you' must die in order for the real you to live. I know that sounds weird, but it is true. That's why the wrong kind of seeking will take you to the wrong path and it sets you on a wrong course.

Feel free to move from any emotion that is God's. A desire to know peace in your heart, wanting to do what is honestly best for your soul; even if it hurts! You want to find your faults because they keep you away from God. You can have honest questions on your heart. What is the Truth? Who is the real you? Whose voices are those other ones that lead you astray? Honest inquisitions for honest answers, all these are okay. If you really genuinely love yourself as God's creation wouldn't you do what is good for you? Who is this other person calling itself 'you' who wants to kill you by deceiving you? This proves that what we know as 'selfishness' is spurred on by demonic spirits and is them in us. Real love always does what is truly good for others, even ourselves.

When you learn how to sit in the presence of Truth, that is when you will begin to know Him and your spirit and chakras will begin to align. But the key is "HE" will do it. The Holy Spirit was sent into the world to lead you and teach you. You cannot assume this position and begin to acquire knowledge out of pride and ambition in order to lead yourself to eternal life. Making an 'I need to fix this' agenda will destroy the effectiveness of the meditation. I know that you have problems and it is very important to you to fix them, but you have to let God do it in His timing and His way. Should you get up in your pride and try to be Him to yourself you will be more lost and ill than ever.

You cannot enter this meditation with a bunch of positive affirmations, aspirations, and lofty goals. What happens when you do this is that you take charge of the healing process instead of Him and a person becomes dependent on the exercise and emotional highs instead of Truth. This is what we want to avoid as it will only deepen your problems. I want you to begin to think of yourself as an extension of God's own character and not separate and not the source of another energy or power. You cannot heal yourself, teach yourself, or originate Truth in any form. Truth is God and you are either in unity with Him or not. You must never see yourself as the Truth itself, but a vessel of Truth. You must meditate each time with a heart that is willing to experience 'whatever' God's Spirit reveals or does not reveal and be willing to see what He wants to show you that day, even if it is nothing. Let your meditation be as natural as possible. Each day will bring differing experiences and moments of truth to your life and will align the chakra points that He deems as necessary. It may be some on each one or a little on one. Each time will differ so begin each mediation with an open mind.

The fact is that only God can align your spirit to His anyway. Any person taking it upon themselves to 'fix' themselves is playing a game of delusion. Let me show it to you in scripture.

22 The light of the body is the eye: if therefore thine eye be single, thy whole body shall be full of light.

23 But if thine eye be evil, thy whole body shall be full of darkness. If therefore the light that is in thee be darkness, how great *is* that darkness!

24 No man can serve two masters: for either he will hate the one, and love the other; or else he will hold to the one, and despise the other. Ye cannot serve God and mammon.

Matt 6:21-24 (KJV)

You are 'serving' someone all the time in whatever you are doing. You can't be served. You can only serve. Did you notice that there are only two sides to choose when it comes to obedience? There is only right and wrong, light and dark. Can you move from a wrong spirit and do the work of God? Whatever emotion you send out, this is the emotion you serve. You will either cling or love the one or the other. This will determine how the chakras align. If you love what is wrong with you how can you separate from it? You can't and it will kill you. The Holy Spirit's challenge is to show you why it is wrong and let you see it for what it really is through inner discovery. If you really want the Truth, He will show it to you. Your heart must want the Truth in order to discover Him.

If your third eye is single, looking for 'one' thing and that is the 'Truth'.....your body will be full of Light. Your chakras will be corrected and healthy.

38 I speak that which I have seen with my Father: and ye do that which ye have seen with your father.

John 8:38 (KJV)

Again, notice that there are only two ways to go, two principals that dictate your life. There is the right way and the wrong way. That's all. You are either on one side of the fence or the other in ever thought and action in your life. If the way you perceive life is through demonic spirits then your spirit dwells in darkness. If your spirit eye is open to the Truth and you are receiving from God who is Truth then your spirit has light. A spirit that dwells in darkness will soon have a body that follows to the dark grave. *In either case you do not originate a way but simply perceive and follow what you perceive. If your perception is incorrect your pathway also becomes incorrect.*

God is the one who tunes your chakras properly. This mistake is made by most who seek to self align their own chakras through so called positive affirmations. None of these affirmations can work when brought from pride and ambition (low frequencies).

There is only One Savior. He must be the one

you sit under to correct your energy points and to align your spirit with His own. Your teacher is Him; the Holy Spirit. Don't look for any answers or try to solve any problems on your own, these will simply unfold as He manifests in you, leading you to the Light. I have seen so many misguided meditations taught to people that I was deeply sickened by them; they don't know how much harm they are doing to people.

Ambition is pride. Pride is of the devil. You must NOT be ambitious in your meditation but only consistent as Daniel was. Your heart must want the Truth and to know Him in you and you must be willing to wait patiently for Him to rescue you from whatever it is that ails you.

Another thing, don't get discouraged with your faults. Everyone begins exactly where they are at—period. The fact that I'm here to write this means I'm not perfectly aligned with the Truth in all things either, so no one has cause to brag. Don't be too eager to share your experiences. People mocking you will greatly discourage you. Let it be a thing that you do in your closet, in the secret of your heart of hearts where you sit down alone with the Father who loves you dearly and you commune and partake in His arms. Keep it intimate and sacred.

Now, there are two positions that work the best for me. The reason that these work the best is because our chakra points are lined up and it creates a better flow of spirit energy.

I want you to go to a quiet room, no distractions.

Using some kind of headphones and the cd are good ways to learn this meditation properly as you follow along with the audio from my website.

Assume a position. I suggest the sitting up one as you can feel your chakra points easily (pg. 250). Choose the one that works best for you. Some people have injured knee joints and so if they sit cross legged it tends to hurt their slightly messed up joints and so if you choose to sit up and you have worn out knees you can put your legs more fully under you placing less stress on your joints and place something under your buttocks to give your body more height.

The main thing you want to accomplish is that your hands must rest palms facing up in a natural manner. You don't want to feel them forced inward or outward. Your fingers should curl naturally and rest without effort facing up on your knees.

The first and most effective position is sitting up with legs crossed and feet under the thighs in the well known meditation position of ancient times. Like I said, if your knees hurt, put your legs underneath more, use a small pillow under your buttocks. I've seen people use phone books or something similar and it works just as well. I like this position because it keeps me alert and I can feel the chakras much stronger than when I lie down. If you can do the meditation this way, you should.

I set up on a pillow if I'm on a soft spot like a bed or mattress in order to not put too much pressure on my knees and pull them under me a bit more then the illustration. Do what works well for you or what feels the most comfortable and natural to you. Then, turn your hands palm up and rest them on your knees to absorb energy from above and close your eyes and tilt your chin slightly downwards. Keep your back fairly straight but do not be rigid. This is the first position.

Again, the public information on chakras and meditation are very misleading and put demons into peoples bodies. Anything that shuts your mind off like chanting and blanking out your mind is an absolute no-no. You want to be fully present and 'awaken' to the Truth, not shut down, in a fixated dream state, or caught up in other thoughts or spirits. Doing so will allow spirits to use your mind and body and teach you to submit to them. This is what most of the meditations do. This is not a good thing and will result in many illnesses and possible demonic possession so please do not do any kind of meditation that teaches you to shut down your own spirit man.

Do not assume the 'lead' position when you meditate. You are following as a sheep does the Shepherd and every time you meditate do it with patience and wait in the moment with anticipation perhaps but more of just a wondering state of mind, attentive, alert. It is important to be fully aware and I will explain how to be in that state in a minute. The point is that you don't want to facilitate demons. Mantras, chants, blanking the mind, and fixations like positive affirmations, music that pulls you into daydreams, and noise are all things you must avoid. You may use natural sounds like birds, water, ocean, or such in a minimal way, perhaps to block road noise or such.....as long as it doesn't cause you to pull into a daydream you are fine.

Before we get into the meditation technique I'm going to cover the next position so you can do whichever you like. The next position which I frequently do is the laying down position and is easier for those who may have bad knees or older folks and also commonly done upon awakening or as one prepares for bed. Lie flat on your back with your arms out comfortably to your side and your palms facing mostly up and your feet slightly apart, put a pillow under just your neck to align your spine and close your eyes. Do not go to sleep. If you feel yourself drifting off, open your eyes, stretch and begin again.

Now, pick a quiet place. You do not want to be interrupted, especially when you are first starting the meditation. Later on, a freight train won't slow you down but it may be a while so don't take on more than your temperament can endure. If you are a mother of little ones this can be difficult, but if you look for times you will often find them during naps and evenings and early mornings. I like sitting in the sunshine in a quiet place or a quiet dark room where oftentimes you can see the brightness of your own aura swirling in colorful patterns of energy.

Basic Overview of the Meditation Process

Okay,......let's begin. Take your position. Either sitting or laying and I prefer you were sitting, begin by **cleansing your temple**. To do this, close your eyes, relax deeply, and then take a deep slow breath. Slowly pull in as much air as you can, swelling out your chest and let it lift your head slightly as you pull it in. Feel the pressure of it. It is as if all your stress, problems, trials, and troubles are within this breath. Pull it all the way to the top or crown of your head, feel your head swell slightly with pressure, it will feel as if it tightens slightly, hold it momentarily......and slowly let it sink to your brow, which is your third eye, you may feel it also swell with an outward pressure, just slightly, then let I slowly move to the base of your throat. You will feel the base of your throat pull inward...now....let it fall down into your chest, your heart will have a sudden sensation of heaviness or pressure.... keep exhaling........ slowly......... and shove the air down into your solar plexus, the place just above your navel...you will feel your stomach sink......continue exhaling and tightening your stomach muscles........ push the air all the way down through your abdomen,...... feel it tighten....continue shoving the air and imagine it exiting out the base of your spine.....tightening your abdomen muscles slightly as needed.....then stop pushing when no air is left in you......and gently inhale a deep slow cleansing breath.....imagine that this is air is **new,** never touched before by any other spirit other than yours and God's. It is sacred space, just between you and Him.

Now...... I want you to relax and begin to inhale and exhale normally. The air that you are now breathing is clean. It is as if you are now breathing heaven's air. (You will find that deep breathing is done instinctively by yourself when you become over stressed and you already instinctively cleanse your soul in this manner in life.)

Now, focus slightly on your hands which are resting gently in an upward position, fingers naturally curled, and resting effortlessly. There is no human being, no one here that can touch you, hurt you, see you, or judge you. It is just you and the Father, no one else is in this space. Notice for a moment that you are alright. All your problems are not you, are they? This is nice to notice.

Now, in your minds eye, notice your fingers on either hand simultaneously, and as you begin to notice them, feel them tingling. Feel the life within them. With your eyes still closed I want you to gaze out into space. Notice that it isn't really dark in there like you had imagined it was before...you never noticed it...perhaps you were too busy or something...but look at it.....there is a light there, a presence with you, this energy is present with you all the time...... I want you to pull the light in through your forehead and let it trickle down through your shoulders into your fingers. Don't strain your eyes, just notice the light and let it wander down into your hands making them grow warm and tingly.

Feel your fingers tingling and your hands growing warmer. There is Life here, coursing through your veins into your hands, you may feel heat in the palms of your hands and pulsating.....just enjoy it.... notice it....feel the Life with you....He is with you....here....in the moment, this is the Father's life giving presence in you, your spirit movement and His, together,...warm and alive....feel Him in you moving, and just enjoy Him. If your whole body tingles let it, and welcome His presence...... feel His life giving energy flowing through you and in you. This is the power that keeps you safe, this presence in your life is here to guide you, He is here right now in you.......welcome Him in again......pull the light in through the center of your forehead, draw it all the way down into your hands ....look for Him and feel Him alive in you.

Feel each finger in turn on each hand, move them slightly if you wish, but let each one tingle and then feel your palms growing warmer and warmer. Feel the light, the warmth, the present moment.

Keep doing this until you find yourself in a daydream. Maybe it was what someone said or did to you. Perhaps a jingle from a commercial or some song....maybe someone said something cruel and made you angry or perhaps it was your to do list, theme music, a show.......whatever it is. Look at the thought that pulled you away from noticing your hands, the warmth of His guiding light until it no longer captures your attention, observe it for a few moments and then pull away from it, and go back to your hands and begin again.

Pull the Light in, feel it coming toward you, invite the light in and let it flow down through you, filtering into your soul and spirit. Let it trickle down your neck, through your arms and into your hands again. At some point you may even experience a tingling sensation that resembles pricking on the top of your head, if you do just enjoy it and continue.....just continue to meditate and enjoy God's presence in you.

Feel the hands tingling and the palms warm again. If you find yourself lost in another thought, pulled away again, don't be angry that you were pulled away. Instead, look at the thought as if it were perhaps on a television in front of your viewing area. Notice the thought and pull gently away and make a choice....do I look at it for awhile or leave? Follow what your heart feels but resist falling into the thought and once you are through go back to your hands, feel the warmth of your palms and look for the Light again, don't strain your eyes, just keep looking and visualizing it coming down your arms into your hands.

If you find that your thoughts overpower you, as will be the case if you are emotionally upset, then oftentimes you are better off to let it run its course and begin again when you have calmed down.

For strong thoughts that seem to persist I take the

sitting position and then imagine that my hands are white light. I observe my hand in my minds eye while lifting one hand slowly to my forehead. I envision the light coming closer and closer to my forehead as I lift my hand slowly and if you do it slowly it will feel as if your hand passes through your head. Its so weird! But it really works to clear your mind from busy noise. Then, do the other hand until your mind is your own again. Be careful not to strain your eyes by over focusing on the light that you see coming at you. I did that a few times by not realizing that I was doing it. So if you notice yourself really pushing your eyes or straining them, just relax them and continue and you'll be fine. This will also tend to open up your third eye.

Once you have your mind back under control start the previous meditation by placing your hands back in to position and begin to feel the hands tingling. Do this over and over, each time a thought pulls you away, look at the thought. You are not your thoughts are you?.....see them out there in front of you causing you grief and going on without you....against your own will....speaking all sorts of nonsense. Pull away from them, feel yourself apart from your thoughts, look at your thoughts, observe, notice them and be aware that you are not your thoughts.

You will find that God will speak to your heart when you begin to pull out of your daydreams and thoughts. You simply have trouble hearing Him due to the large volume of noise going on in your head.

Stand every 15 to 20 minutes and stretch. The main stretch I want you to do is one that will surprise you. Stand up, raise your hands above your head and reach up, extending your arms high into the air. Then, slowly lower both of your arms extending them fully, outward away from your body like you were an airplane and continue lowering them all the way to your side. If you are paying attention, as you slowly lower your arms you will feel each chakra point as your arms come all the way down to your side. Do you feel like more? If you do, continue.

Try to meditate as often as three times a day. Morning is most crucial. If you feel like doing more meditation, like a stirring in your soul, then proceed. If not, stretch really good and go about your day. It is that simple. Most of your revelations will come during the day. Why? You are learning to pull out of your thoughts and hear God in your spirit.

Let God do the work in you, you just come to the Light with a pure heart to see the truth because you want it. I suggest 15 minutes of tongues between the silent meditation. Pray in tongues from the meditation position. You may find yourself swaying during tongues, bowing, crying, or such...whatever the case, follow along without giving thought to it. Let it flow naturally from you. You belong the Him and as you are coming from a correct place in your heart, He will meet with you and your meditations will be blessed by Him.

Use my meditation audio file to help you begin

but continue on your own when it starts to become repetitive to you. You must hear God in you, not me.

I also recommend that you speak in tongues during the day while doing things like mowing, dishes, and daily chores. Ideally we should pray an hour a day in tongues. Tongues is an open dialogue between you and the Father and emits high frequencies. It is your spirit, chakras, beseeching His and aligning. You can sit in the same position, envision the Light and pray with your palms up, feeling your fingers tingle while you pray. This will keep your mind in the present. It has been proven by science that part of your frontal lobe shuts down during tongues speech. I believe that this is because your spirit is emitting high frequencies in accordance with His from your chakras.

Alternate between tongues and silence but let each meditation take its course and be an adventure unto itself. Eventually you can pray in tongues in silence. You will hear it in your spirit in your mind's eye just like you do you own voice or the voice of other spirits in you. We are amazing beings, creatures really in Christ Jesus.

Don't use music in your meditation. You don't want to drift off into a dream state of the great bygone days or the wondrous days to come or the 'how could she do that to me' thoughts or 'look how awesome I am now' thoughts. You want to pull away from the dream stuff and find God in Reality. Again, the blessings generally come after the meditation because what you are learning to do is to be present in the here and now of every day life. You will begin to see things as they really are and demons will begin to find it impossible to get you to emit low frequencies! You will begin to notice things about yourself and others that you weren't able to see before and pull out of the deception of every day life.

Things will begin to be very apparent as you move from the darkness into the Light. You will see why people use you, why you use other, and in this awareness, obedience comes, and from obedience you will begin to find unity with God. From unity with God you will begin to experience Him through revelations, sensations, concepts, and the power to really live unto Him and He will move through you. High frequencies will begin to pulsate from your being, you will find angels by your side, and the kingdom of heaven will be your dwelling place.

This world will begin to become a more defined place as you now able to make the right choices, follow the right paths, and do that which is correct. You will feel joy as your Father approves of you, peace comes and guilt becomes a thing of the past, and the more you move upon, the more He will give to you. For you have been a good and faithful steward of all that He has blessed you with instead of the person who became clouded by the voices in his mind, losing what had been given to him by His Father amongst the confusion.

What does a perfect chakra look like? Jesus' of course! He is the Way, the Truth, and the Life. That is why He came. Jesus never emitted even one low frequency. He was without sin.

A perfect person is one who does not offend the Truth in what they do.

1 My brethren, be not many masters, knowing that we shall receive the greater condemnation.

2 For in many things we offend all. If any man offend not in word, the same is a perfect man, and able also to bridle the whole body.
                                        James 3:1-2 (KJV)

A sign that things are beginning to take affect is a mouth that aligns and begins to speak from the abundance of a pure heart. *If any man offend not in word, the same is a perfect man.* Your mouth will show you where your heart is at. What is coming out of your mouth? Do you speak words of doubt or fear? Are you condemning or criticizing? This meditation exercise will allow you to actually observe what is taking place in your life.

James was not talking about offending people or hurting people's feelings as some misinterpret this scripture, but offending God and speaking out against Him and His ways. If you don't 'offend' the truth in you.....you are also able to bridle your whole body. If you can live and not ever move against or contrary to Him, then you are a perfect soul. It was just a statement of Truth. In verse eight we see the truth of the matter....no human being can tame the tongue. Only the Truth revealed to the inner man can make a soul perfect. Only the Truth accepted in the inner man can tame the tongue.

8 But the tongue can no man tame; *it is* **an unruly evil, full of deadly poison.**

How does an evil tongue effect you? It can and will destroy your life. Only God can correct your spirit....you cannot. Be humble, see the Truth, and in your contrition you will find your Father.

May your journey on this planet be one of Truth and may I some day meet you with His light shining strong in your eyes. Soon we will see the Truth as He is and all those who adore the Truth will be with Him....forever. Therefore, make ready your garments and seek the truth while He can be found. For all who love the ways of darkness, those who hate the light of their own conscience, these will be destroyed by the brightness of His coming. May you not be named among them.

"For with thee is the fountain of life: in thy light shall we see light"
Psalms 36:9 (KJV)

www.ingramcontent.com/pod-product-compliance
Lightning Source LLC
LaVergne TN
LVHW051449080426
835509LV00017B/1712